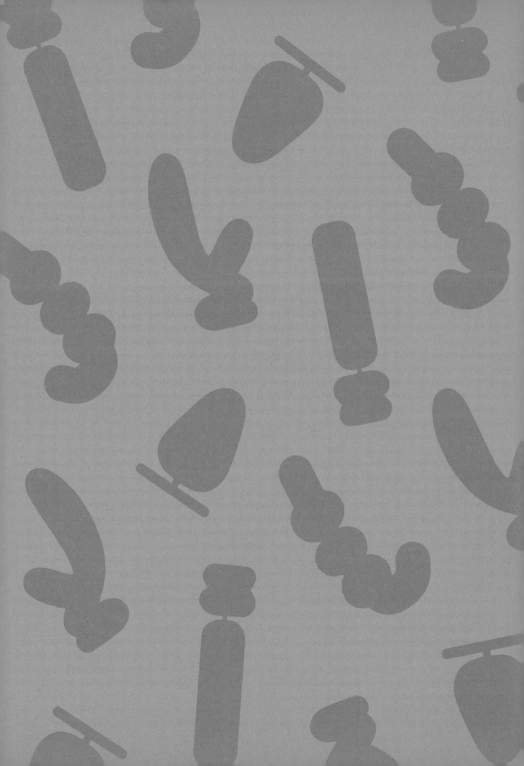

MY
PLEASURE

MY
PLEA

AN INTIMATE GUIDE TO
LOVING YOUR BODY AND
HAVING GREAT SEX

by LAURA DELARATO
illustrations by Amber Vittoria

SURE

CHRONICLE BOOKS
SAN FRANCISCO

Library of Congress Cataloging-in-Publication Data
Names: Delarato, Laura, author. I Vittoria, Amber, illustrator.
Title: My pleasure : an intimate guide to loving your body and having great sex / by Laura Delarato ; illustrated by Amber Vittoria.
Description: San Francisco : Chronicle Books, [2022]
Identifiers: LCCN 2021027970 I ISBN 9781797210742 (hardcover)
Subjects: LCSH: Sex instruction. I Sexual excitement. I Self-acceptance.I Masturbation.
Classification: LCC HQ56 .D326 2022 I DDC 613.9071--dc23
LC record available at https://lccn.loc.gov/2021027970

Manufactured in China.

Design by Rachel Harrell.

Edited by Claire Gilhuly and Sydney Fowler.

Typesetting by Kelly Abeln.

10 9 8 7 6 5 4 3 2 1

Chronicle Books LLC
680 Second Street
San Francisco, California 94107
www.chroniclebooks.com

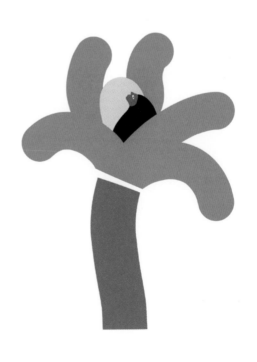

TABLE OF CONTENTS

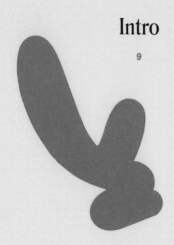
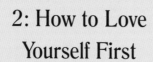
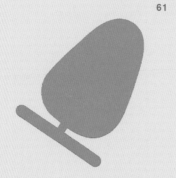

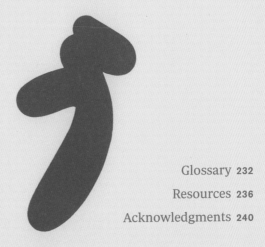

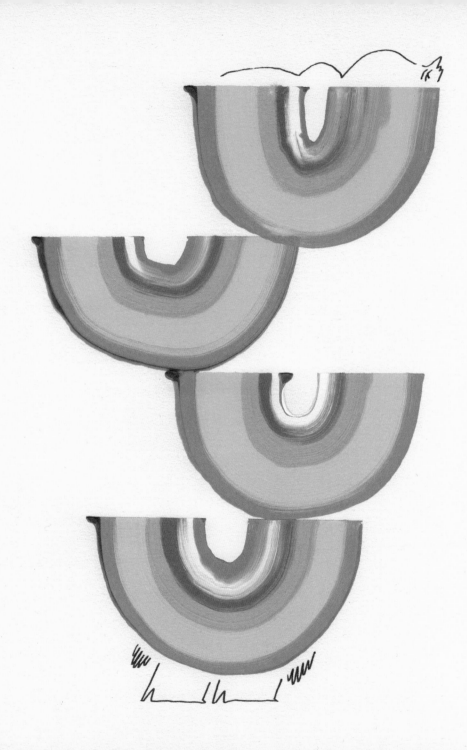

Intro

Pleasure.

'ple-zhər, a state
of gratification, a
sensual joy, a frivolous
amusement. The
sensation when
something feels good.

There are plenty of ways to define the word *pleasure*. We all know what it is, but the practical application of pleasure is a lesson we glossed over on our way to developing nerve endings, sex organs, wet dreams, boners, hard nipples, and, of course, masturbating against the high-pressure shower spray (a favorite). We develop, we're taught through any means we can find (old *Playboys* for me), and then one day we find we are adults with a sex life in which we're not able to ask a partner to swirl their tongue the way we want them to.

THINGS I LEARNED IN HIGH SCHOOL SEX ED

- Women who put on too much makeup are asking for it.

- Boys will be boys.

- "Time of the month" is how you respectfully talk about menstruation.

- Sex is just for making babies.

- Contracting an STI means you're dirty.

- Condoms are unnecessary because pregnancy is something the girls want and STIs are impossible if you are monogamous.

- Being aroused just means you need to exercise [eye roll].

- The pill makes you unattractive and messes up your hormones for life.

- Marital rape is impossible.

- Blue balls are very dangerous, so if you say you're having sex, you need to follow through.

- NOTE: None of this is true.

- ANOTHER NOTE: All of this is garbage.

- ANOTHER ANOTHER NOTE: We all deserve a lot better than this.

Also, hi. I'm Laura. I'll be the one guiding you through this book I've written about the abundant glory that is sexual pleasure and its positive effects on every aspect of your life.

My teen self is shocked that adult me is writing this book for you. Well, actually, I'm not *that* surprised that I spent a ton of time researching and categorizing sex toys (get ready for chapter 4, babes). Mainly, I'm shocked that, with my collective history as a struggling, plus-size person, I found a way through it all to become an expert on the subject. But mostly, I feel really proud that this book gets to be both something for you in your pleasure and body-love journey and something that culminates years of working on my own experience for me.

My relationship to my body and pleasure starts around age twelve, when I grew boobs, got my period, shot up to around five foot seven, and developed hips and a belly that pressed against my Spice Girls T-shirts. I felt like a monster—fully over-grown and an incredible sore thumb compared to the rest of my peers. My body looked more mature than I was ready for, and the attention given to me was simultaneously painful and confusing. I was being praised for having boobs by men twice my age—something I thought, at the time, was my only output into the world—while being told my body was a disgusting, excessive bag of period blood, sweat, acne, and blubber by magazines, TV shows, every single movie, family members, and every peer that happened to be thin enough to shop at Fashion Bug while I browsed the accessories. I was Ursula. I was Fat Monica. I was every chubby girl who made an excuse to not go to the pool party. I was the sidekick and never the love interest.

It didn't help that my childhood was a wishy-washy world of instability as I went back and forth between my Italian grandparents' house in the Bronx, where they would withhold pasta from my plate because I was too chubby, and my mother's house in Virginia, where she drank more than she ate, and refused to let me be anything other than a kid on a diet. In fact, I don't remember a moment during that time where I wasn't trying to find ways to be smaller. I remember going into a dressing room with my mother when I was twelve as she tried to squeeze me into a skirt much smaller than my preteen body, and exclaiming for the entire dressing room to hear: "Laura, you've got to lose some of this weight." My weight was a constant problem for everyone else—even for my younger brother, who one day during the summer brought me outside to our concrete backyard in the Bronx and insisted I do sprints so that he didn't go to high school with a fat sister.

Honestly, I don't blame them. Not because they were right . . . they weren't. But because they were doing what they thought was right. None of us were taught to love ourselves. None of us understood the impacts of negative self-image. None of us had the language to express the connection between loving your body and experiencing pleasure. And as a result, from that point, I desperately wanted to be thin. I spent ages twelve to twenty-six as an on-again-off-again bulimic with a tendency toward crash dieting, Weight Watchers, and phentermine— and it bled into my adult life. As a kid, I would brush it off like there was something wrong with me, but as an adult I have found myself distrusting others who show me affection, feeling like I don't deserve pleasure, and being at a full-blown war with my body when I'm hungry.

THINGS TOLD TO ME BY DOCTORS ABOUT MY WEIGHT

- "Maybe if you laid off the candy, you would lose weight and that cough would go away." —age 13

- "To be healthy, you need to starve yourself." —age 18

- "If you strive for 1 pound a week, you'll be 10 pounds thinner before school starts in the fall." —age 20

- "I don't have to tell you that you don't look very healthy, right?" —age 26

Did sixteen-year-old Laura know that adult Laura would be sitting at her desk most nights telling people to love themselves? No. She was too entangled in a chaotic environment, being swallowed by her own eating disorder, to ever think she'd make it through college. She was dyeing her hair green with Kool-Aid and trying to match her voice to the monotone stylings of Daria. She wasn't applying herself because she didn't think she had anything to offer.

Right around the age of twenty-five, I was living in a shoebox in Brooklyn and paying $500 in rent with four other roommates and a dog. I was getting my master's degree in media and production at The New School in the West Village and freelancing at night at MTV2. It was this serendipitous moment in my life, when I needed a job close to school so I could easily pick up shifts to pay my rent and continue to take classes, that I found a job at the famous sex toy store, the Pleasure Chest. The Pleasure Chest looked like a fun place to spend time that didn't involve school or production sheets or four roommates and a dog (though I do love dogs). It was a bit of a safe haven for me—a place where I got to learn about pleasure for all bodies and people, a place where it wasn't weird to ask questions.

At the Pleasure Chest, I read every book on the shelves, watched every porn video, learned about every product, and understood what it meant to be body positive, sex positive, and confident, but I still didn't know how to put it into action for myself.

Then, everything changed. I was invited to a drink-and-draw class at a plus-size vintage store in downtown Brooklyn. I still remember walking in, finding a seat with my art supplies, and being totally struck by the model, a fat, queer dream who owned the platform they stood on—fully nude and covered in pearls, feathers, and bright red lipstick. A self-identified fat person who didn't care if the position of their body or the fullness of their size was seen as disruptive by popular society. It was that moment when I realized everything in my life needed to be different. I remember saying to myself: *This is no way to live. This is a way to die.*

Even after that point, it took me a really long time to discover that my body wasn't a problem. That there wasn't a thin woman dying to come out so I could start my life. No matter how much weight I lost or how many times I went to the gym, it didn't matter if I didn't learn to love and accept myself from the inside out. The confidence it takes to make decisions

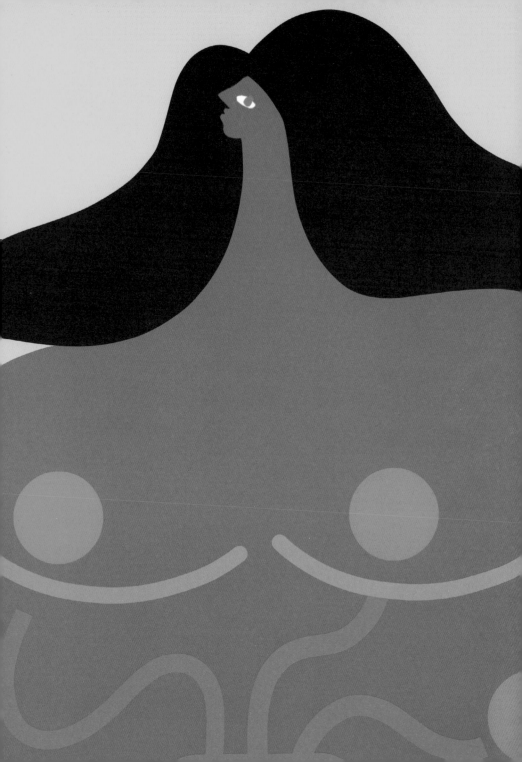

based on your own needs, wear the clothing you want to wear, feel comfortable with your naked body, or even jump on top of your partner without concern over cellulite or belly rolls has nothing to do with losing weight or "fixing" yourself to match a beauty standard. You can't buy confidence at the grocery store. You have to confront what you've learned, smash it, and rebuild a better foundation. And that foundation of body love, acceptance, and confidence, my dear reader, is essential to a healthy sex life.

MY IDEAL GROCERY STORE

- There would be diverse images in each aisle.

- *Fat-free* would be taken off every package.

- The person with the samples would hand out an array of options that suits your hunger at that moment.

- Flyers for therapy and self-help groups would be on prominent display for anyone struggling with body image or dysmorphia.

- There would be zero GMOs, artificial sweeteners, pesticides, or harmful preservatives that involuntarily heighten or crash your mood.

- Cashiers would remind you that you're royalty and deserve the best this world has to offer.

This book is dedicated to that moment where you, me, all of us realize we deserve the best this life has to offer. *My Pleasure* is about celebrating positive body image and personal pleasure in order to achieve an amazing solo and partnered sex life. This book will be one part deeply explorative—it will reconnect you to how you feel about your body and help you think positively about your body—and the other part serviceable—each chapter includes activities and actionable ways to find pleasure by yourself and/or with a partner(s). Throughout it all, I will be here, guiding the way and sharing fun tidbits from my own life—and sex life!

So now we're here. What's next? Well, reading a book about pleasure in various forms is deeply intimate—almost like getting to know someone. You could even say we're BFFs! And because we've entered into this book relationship, we're going to get to know each other pretty intimately over the next two-hundred-some-odd pages. But first, let me tell you what I'm bringing to the table.

I'm a body image and sexual wellness advocate, working and writing in the industry for the last ten years (which is honestly so wild to think about!). I'm a Pisces, which apparently means something

HOT TIP

THE MY PLEASURE CODE

When you feel good about your body, you feel good about your choices. And when you feel good about your choices, you can feel good about your pleasure.

really cool according to all the apps that send me mystical notifications. When I get a haircut, I always base it on an era—I've been living in the '90s for quite a while now. I have a bachelor's degree in English journalism and a master's degree in media studies—but honestly, does that even matter anymore? I have an absurd amount of art supplies. And, I've always loved books that break away from the words and check in on the reader. *Hello, how are you? Do we need a sip of water for this part?* You'll find that a lot of what I do in this book is present an idea that you can apply to your life, and then check in with what's going on with you.

When I was given the opportunity to write this book, I thought long and hard (lol) about how I wanted this book to read, how I wanted people to use it, how I wanted each paragraph and chapter to sound the moment it was finished. While it is a guidebook of sorts, my hope is that this book is also fun to read and to use. After all, it is literally all about your pleasure . . . well, *My Pleasure*, but you get the point. We'll break down why pleasure is so important, why you deserve it, and the many ways to get it (and to get off). Sometimes you need someone to champion you—let me (and this book) do that for you!

Before we go down this road together and form a bond through words and pages, here are some things to expect from me and this book—and what I expect from you.

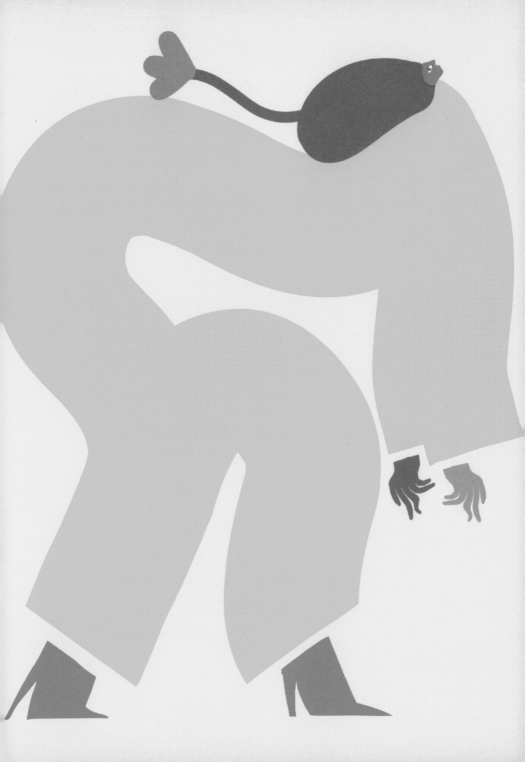

WHAT TO EXPECT FROM ME

- I love every punny bit of ridiculousness that comes with writing anything about bodies and sex and vulvae and penises.

- But! Even with the puns, you can expect me to be conscious of gender, identity, and pronouns throughout the book. It's important to me that anyone and everyone (people who identify as queer or straight, people who are transgender or cisgender or gender nonconforming, people of size, people who don't identify with plus-size, people from all racial backgrounds, people with different levels of ability, people from different social and economic backgrounds) can find themselves within these pages.

- I'm not always going to know all the answers, but I will do my best to help you figure them out.

- I have a fairly sunny disposition in contrast with some real moments. If I can impart one lesson right at the top, it would be that not every day is going to be a good body image day.

WHAT I EXPECT FROM YOU

- Modify what you need. You don't have to jump right into an activity or adopt advice if it's uncomfortable.

All I ask is that you take a moment to question that discomfort and where it comes from.

- Be honest with yourself. Does it feel good to do XYZ? If not, why not?

- Contradictions will happen—the world is filled with them. It's OK to feel one way about one thing and another way about another thing. Give yourself room to grow and form a personal, well-thought-out opinion.

- No settling. If you're going to do something, let it be grand.

- Hold space for yourself to find what you need from this book.

- If you don't know an answer, that's OK! You can always come back to it.

After so many years of being at war with my body and finding it difficult to experience pleasure in so many ways, I dedicated my entire soul to being an authority on the subject of pleasure to anyone who would listen to me. Welcome to *My Pleasure*, babes. This one's for you.

GETTING TO KNOW YOU

Like I said, use this book in whatever way you need. If you want to take notes, skip around, jump ahead, or even start your own little companion notebook to use with the exercises, be my guest! For right now, just get to know a bit about who you are so that you never stray from yourself throughout the journey. Following are some questions. Find a relaxing space with a beverage (may I suggest a peppermint tea with lemon—my favorite) and take some time to get to know yourself.

- What is your name?

- Do you love your name? Why or why not?

- Where are you from?

- What are some activities you like to do that make you feel happy?

- Is there a person or character you really identify with? Why?

- Who are the people or characters you most admire and why?

- Who in your life doesn't make you feel great? How so?

- When was the last time someone made you uncomfortable? What happened?

- Describe a meal, any meal that makes you feel good. It can be an elaborate one!

- What era do you love the most? Why?

- When was the last time you felt sexy? What was happening?

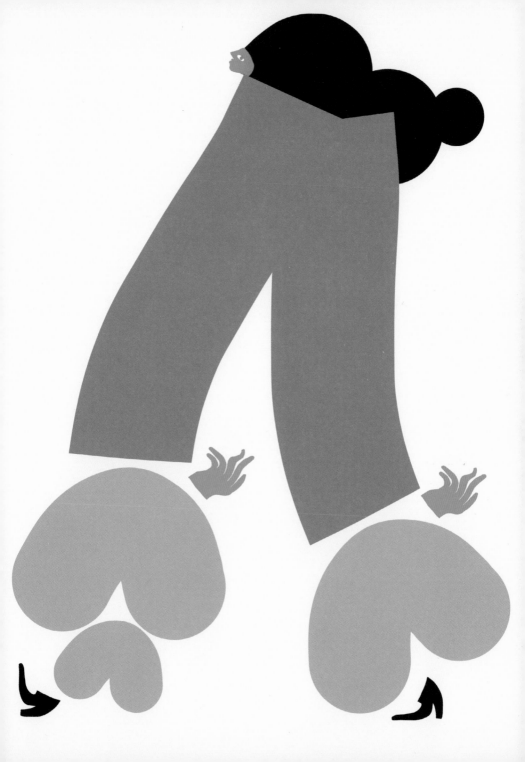

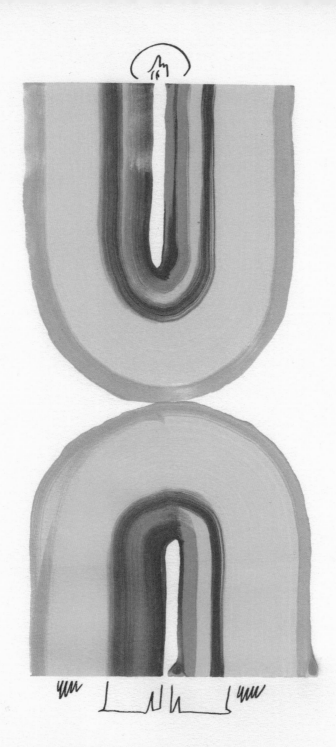

1

Welcome

to Your

Body

Hello, good morning,
good afternoon,
good day.

Welcome to chapter
numero uno, where we
start this bad boy and
get down to the nitty
gritty of pleasure, self-
love, and great sex.

First off, if you were expecting a book where we go over the hottest sex positions and the best ways to please your partner, sorry to tell you . . . this isn't it. Let me redirect you to another book aisle. If you're still with me—and I hope you are!—this book is very much intended to get at the root of YOUR pleasure, and believe it or not, that all comes from within. And while I LOVE a sex position chat or a how-to on doing that little thing with your tongue to send them over the edge, my top priority is for you to love your body and live a pleasurable life (which, in turn, will give you the confidence to try those sexual techniques and positions with more self-assurance). First, we have to connect with ourselves and learn to love our quirks; the hot sex and self-love will follow.

As much as I want to say, "Do these 5 things to achieve maximum pleasure," I have to be honest: It takes a lot of mental work, some unlearning and relearning, and some trust before we can really love ourselves fully and thus experience uninhibited pleasure—and that's OK! There are going to be bad days, awful days, days in which seeking self-love in any form is going to feel like a waste of time. But I promise, no matter how comfortable it is to hate ourselves (as we've been trained to do), it's so much brighter on the other side, even on a cloudy day.

WHAT'S YOUR STORY?

Our bodies are so interesting and weird and exciting and soft. A vessel that moves us from place to place. An ever-changing figure that inherits specific genetic traits from our family line. A frame that we maintain and take care of when it's sick or hurt or run-down. Our bodies hold our memories too—any experienced microaggressions, traumas, pleasures, and joys. They are a blueprint of our lives. As we get older, we grow and mature, but our past has an interesting way of worming into our present and affecting our self-image, and it's helpful to be aware of that. Every single time we get naked, are intimate, connect with ourselves, or trust others, we are laying bare our insecurities and self-confidence. Our personal history creates a conscious (and a lot of times, unconscious) rubric for how we handle everything—especially our sex lives and our self-love. When we don't know our history or our triggers, it's significantly more difficult to embrace who we are and what we want and to make considerate and smart decisions. Let's take a moment to reflect on our story and identify what bothers us, what triggers us, and what sends us down a negative path. Then, taking all of that into account, let's devise an action plan to take care of ourselves.

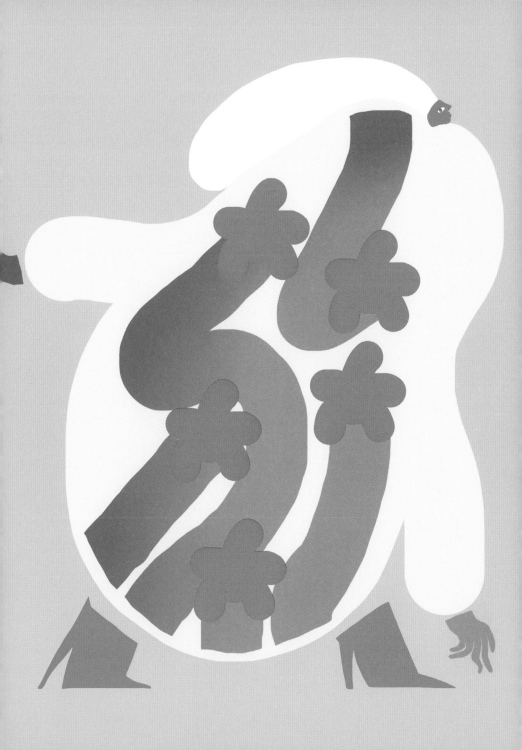

THE LIFE STORY MAP

If I were to ask you to write out the bullet points of your life story, what would that list look like? What are the particular memories and moments that have created, changed, or disrupted the person you are today? Basically, what were the key milestones that built you? The list can be as serious or as fun as you make it, as long as it comes from an honest place—but spend no more than 15 minutes on the subject and maybe plan to do something kind for yourself afterward! While this can be a really intriguing exercise to understand your life story, it can also bring up some traumatic memories for some, and we certainly want to refrain from getting sucked into that sensory detail. Take this short time to write out those bullet points in your life.

To know thyself is to love thyself, and we're on a mission to be self-loving.

WHO WERE YOU AS A KID?

We are the past, present, and future versions of ourselves in every single moment of our lives. Looking at our lives holistically like this can help explain our reactions and feelings in any given situation. Even if our emotional maturity is at an all-time high, the childish versions of ourselves can come out when we get overwhelmed, caught off guard, scared, or frustrated.

Next time you get upset, take note of the emotions, actions, and reactions that come through when your guard is down. Got 'em? Great. Write them down! Here are some of mine.

- I stomp my feet when I get frustrated . . . I'm a woman in my thirties. Cool cool cool.

- I will tear up when I get overwhelmed. My therapist says this is because I never had a childhood and didn't develop good coping mechanisms . . . pshhh, whatever :::tears:::

- My first reaction is to be very mean when someone crosses me . . . kind of like a kid on a playground. See previous.

Got your list? Perfect. Now we can start to look for patterns when those feelings show up. For the next week or two, every time you feel these feelings, take note of when they occur and why. What causes these feelings to surface? You can even input each entry into a calendar (if you're like me, the calendar is fully color-coded). After keeping track for a period of time, see if you can spot any connections. Maybe you hadn't eaten when those reactions happened. Maybe it was after a difficult conversation with a family member. Maybe you were simply tired. But now you know, and you can better counteract those reactions with data. Think of this as getting to know yourself on a deeper, more intimate level.

We all want to be hot babes living as our truest selves, asking for what we want, getting what we deserve, and accomplishing our dreams, all while having earth-shattering orgasms. Yes to all of this. But we must consider our backstory—not because we can't have all that good stuff without a particular backstory—not at all. Rather, because who we are, how we act, and how we feel about ourselves and our bodies is shaped by those rise-to-the-occasion moments in our past.

- EXHIBIT A: Adults who had negative experiences in their childhood—from peer bullying to their parents' divorce to exposure to aggressive adult figures—have higher anxiety, lower understanding of their needs, and a greater likelihood of unsatisfying sex.

- EXHIBIT B: Childhood neglect has long-term effects on adulthood, making it difficult to trust others, stay connected, and ask for what we need.

- EXHIBIT C: Adolescent and childhood dieting take a huge mental toll on a developing brain. Teaching kids to control their appearance leads to disordered eating, food guilt, and poor self-worth and self-esteem.

You get the point. Even if you didn't experience this severity of trauma in your childhood, we all have negative lived experiences that imprint on our brains. And after all that, we still think we can just go on our merry way and "BE CONFIDENT" and start developing our own sense of pleasure and acceptance and excellent sex lives without considering what has been impacted in the process. Unfortunately, it's not that easy. We first have to come to terms with our story and make the necessary changes to our perspectives in order to get us to a better mental place where we can love ourselves.

How to Process I'm not a doctor or therapist or someone who collects data. But I'm fairly certain if you're a person who is breathing, you have experienced some form of suffering. Consider collective trauma: Hello, COVID-19. These kinds of difficult experiences manifest in different ways in each of us and can cause both physical and mental harm when left unprocessed.

The negative impact of these experiences isn't just "in your head." They can leave an imprint on your body and/or your brain, which is why it's really important for you to find the best way to feel mentally sound. Therapy is great; telehealth is fantastic. Finding groups, taking prescribed medication, having a list of people to talk to, taking walks, journaling, practicing yoga, creating spiritual rituals, and soaking in some vitamin D can help you process your past so you can freely live your future.

Recognizing Your Emotional Triggers Identify topics or people who make you feel uncomfortable:

- Are there people or social media accounts that you compare yourself to? Why? What is that internal conversation like? Sure, you can unfollow the account, but we want to get to the heart of why it makes you feel uncomfortable, so you have that reference for yourself.

- Let's say a friend has some great news to share. You're super happy but you're feeling very "Why not me?" about it. What is the news? In other words, what are the topics that can make you feel a bit emotional and intense?

Rethink, Revise, Rewrite for the Future

The past is the past is the past and there is nothing we can do about our lived experiences. What we can do is go for better next time. Here are a few ways we can learn from the past so we can live better in the future.

1| Reflect, but don't obsess. Give yourself a short time limit to engage in that reflection.

2| Study the moment, but try not to judge.

3| Take someone else's position. In the heat of the moment, it's impossible to see anyone else's point of view. Once you have some distance, try to reflect on the experience, without judgment, from another POV.

4| Remember it and release it. That moment will always be etched in your memory, but the associated emotions don't have to be. Write the memory on a piece of paper, say it out loud, then burn it (safely) while repeating, "I will no longer hold on to this memory" until the paper is fully incinerated. (I typically do this in a sink and turn the water on immediately once the paper is burned, just to be safe!)

5| Reframe the circumstance and use it for the future. Was this a necessary learning experience in order to be your better future self? None of us is perfect or going to feel perfect all the time, and forgiving yourself for past mistakes is an excellent way to add more self-love into your life.

REFLECT AND REFRAME

I'd love for you, dear reader, to use the preceding 5 steps as a way to reflect on a not-so-positive experience from your past. Write it down in your notebook or on the facing page, and see if you can find something positive in it. And just so you don't feel weird doing this, here is mine.

- **REFLECT:** I was in an open relationship—an intimate connection that is sexually nonmonogamous—that required me to tell my primary partner when I slept with another person. But I didn't do that. Instead, when I slept with someone else, I covered it up and lied about it. A year later, when the lie came out, my primary partner was angry, rightly so, and it led to the end of our relationship.

- **STUDY:** There are parts of me that still want to justify my actions, but in truth, I made poor choices that had negative consequences.

- **NEW POV:** That person probably felt lied to, stupid, and untrusted in our relationship. I would have felt the same way.

- **RELEASE IT:** It's been some time. I've apologized, I've tried to be more honest, I've acknowledged where I need to improve. I will always carry it with me, but for now I need to move forward and use what I have learned about myself to have better relationships.

- **REFRAME AND USE IT:** In hindsight, I realize I wasn't being honest with myself and what I wanted. In the future, I need to be more mindful of my feelings and 100 percent true to who I am.

- **NOW, YOU TRY.**
  Reflect:
  Study:
  New POV:
  Release It:
  Reframe and Use It:

KNOWING YOUR OWN WORTH

Why, hello there, you worthy, cool human, you! Did you know that you deserve a five-course-meal type of life with a tasty starter, excellent conversation, water breaks, and all the refills that your body desires? Yes, you! Self-worth is a tricky thing that is deeply connected to how we interact, engage, and treat others and ourselves. And it's about time we recognized just how amazing we really are. But to do that, we need to work on our self-esteem. As we move forward, just know that you deserve all the goodness this life has to offer!

Self-Esteem and External Messaging

Now that we've looked into our past, we're going to turn to our present. Consider the messaging that's happening all around you, all the time—from the media, your social circle, and your social media. Even if you're not consciously consuming it, you are absorbing these messages that contribute to your self-worth.

Self-worth is a tricky thing. We inherently understand that we are good people who deserve to be treated with respect, but there are hidden messages in everything we do and everything we experience that often tell us otherwise.

WHERE WE SEE THESE MESSAGES

I grew up to be a plus-size babe with a larger belly than most. This shouldn't take away my value in the world. I've been this way my whole life, and according to 23andMe (or any other genealogy/ancestry mapping website), this is just the way it is! Might as well love it, right? But there are so many messages I face all day that tell me that my value is lesser because of my personal facts. Maybe you experience this as well?

- I can't find clothes in stores.

- Most clothes I like aren't available in my size.

- Representations of me and my body are often parodied.

- I can't walk down the street without someone making a fat joke.

- Every piece of advice I get is about weight loss.

- Every Tinder message I get is "I love big girls."

And it's not just me:

- The internet hates fat people . . . we already know that.

- Plus-size women make less money because of size bias.

- Plus-size women are less likely to be believed in a sexual harassment case.

- Plus-size women are less likely to be hired.

And to top it all off, I can't even get a consultation for Invisalign without being told that one of the benefits is that people lose weight because they eat less with them!

Have these and other things changed the way I view myself? Yes. Of course they have. We forget that there are entire corporations and industries designed to teach us what is right and wrong. Living through body negativity is like breathing in pollution: The more we're exposed, the worse it is on our health, and it's often impossible to avoid. This makes it really difficult to stop believing these messages.

When we're faced with such a wild amount of disdain at the hands of the entire universe, we try to change, to be amicable, to make ourselves as small as possible. This can lower our self-esteem. It also makes it really easy for us to make bad decisions about our bodies, and for others to take advantage of us.

QUESTION TIME

- Have you ever gone out of your way to do something simply to receive acknowledgment or a low reward from another person?

- Do you feel like you'll be dismissed if you don't give 110 percent of yourself to friends, lovers, or even people you barely know?

- Have you ever felt like you had to perform a sexual act to be liked or admired, to feel beautiful or worthy?

Oh darlings, it's not enough to just be a human in this world. We have to deal with the complexities of how we internalize our value based on the information we've learned and the messaging we've been exposed to. Who here isn't guilty of feeling less? Who hasn't thought if they simply became a new person, life would be better?

SIGNS OF LOW SELF-ESTEEM

- Difficulty prioritizing one's needs

- Saying sorry for everyday slipups

- Not feeling deserving of happiness

- Trouble making and standing by choices

- Lack of boundaries

- Buying excessive gifts for other people

- Negative self-perception

- Abusive internal dialogue

Know Your Worth Casual sex friends can be a wonderful thing, but you have to know where to draw the line! There was a time when I was seeing a person who kept pushing back the time of our sex date. And finally I got a text that read: "Hey, want to come over at eleven?" There I was walking to this person's house late at night. It hit me: *What do I actually want to be doing right now?* I texted the person, "Hey, I'm tired. Let's hang when it's a good time for both of us," turned around, bought a burrito, and went home. Nothing about the scenario made me feel good or even want to engage. I said yes because I thought that was what I was supposed to do if someone was (vaguely) interested in me. We never saw each other after that, which feels appropriate. No one deserves to be strung along by a person who can't commit to a reasonable hour.

Now my answer to an 11 p.m. date is: I'm an adult with an adult job, so nah.

You see, knowing and valuing who you are is how self-love and pleasure happen.

Self-esteem is the building block of autonomy. If you know yourself mentally and physically, and respect yourself, you're more likely to make good decisions for your brain and body (such as not going on dates when you're tired, not putting yourself second, recognizing that a burrito might be more pleasurable than a booty call in certain moments. See preceding). So, how exactly do we develop self-esteem?

Embrace Yourself

All I want to tell you is that you're the best and send you on your hot, merry way. But the issue here is—and I'm sure you've experienced this—no matter what I say or what anyone else says, you have to believe it yourself as well. Isn't that just absurd? I would have so much confidence if my brain truly believed all the positive things my friends and family say to me. But my brain refuses to accept it. So, how do we work on this?

It may be difficult, but the next time someone compliments you, simply say, "Thank you." You don't have to believe it or do anything with that information. All you have to do is acknowledge the person with those two words. Over time, this will get easier and easier, and eventually—hopefully—you might actually believe them. Once we accept the idea that we are deserving, it's so much easier to face criticism, deal with difficult moments, and still feel good about ourselves at the end of the day. Accepting a compliment is a good first step.

How else can we value ourselves? How can we find our way to self-acceptance? Here, I've listed my 10 Commandments for embracing who we are. Take your time with each, go slow, and find yourself on the other side.

THE 10 COMMANDMENTS OF EMBRACING YOURSELF

1| GET TO KNOW YOURSELF. We're learning our story, we're coming to terms with who we are, we're tackling our most uncomfortable pieces of history . . . we're on our way to full acknowledgment!

2| RECONSIDER SELF-CRITIQUES. Look, sometimes you're going to have to face yourself and say, "Babe, that wasn't great." But be gentle. When we criticize ourselves, it can send us on a spiral of other things we consider wrong about ourselves. People with marginalized identities often internalize false beliefs about their communities, leading to negative beliefs about themselves. It's important when we get in that spiral to recognize that these personal critiques are not only wrong but also reinforce oppressive systems. Sure, I can say, "Breathe in, let go as you breathe out, and move toward empathy with yourself." Maybe that can help, if only momentarily. But it's also important to be critical of those self-critiques when they arise.

3| LOOK TOWARD THE POSITIVE. I know we're all used to preparing for the worst, but your worst days might all be behind you. What if you started thinking that good things will happen?

4| CHAMPION SUCCESSES. Make a cool portfolio or zine or resume or art piece dedicated to your coolness.

Personal projects are a great way to ritualize self-love. Success for you could also look like survival or resistance to external or internalized oppression. Acknowledge and champion your existence in your own way.

5| TONE DOWN WORRYING. Chances are, you're the only one worried about this one particular thing. Ask yourself: What is the return on investment (ROI) of worrying about this issue? (A little business lingo for ya!) If you can't justify the stress, then drink some tea and calmly say goodbye to it in your head.

6| BUT DO ACKNOWLEDGE STRESS. When we let stress run around our bodies, it can really drain us emotionally. Rather than pushing whatever it is that's stressing you out to the back burner, write it down, make a to-do list, and prioritize. Acknowledge it and take action.

7| FORGIVE YOURSELF. We're all going to make mistakes. We're human, and it's part of the deal, ya know? Consider that the reason mistakes happen is so you can learn that lesson for the future. Mistakes are mini classes that help us gain emotional resiliency for whatever life throws at us.

8| PRACTICE GRATITUDE. You're here working on yourself, looking for a better route to sexual pleasure and body love—give yourself some grace and gratitude for being here right now.

9| LOOK AT YOUR BODY ... A LOT. Guess what? You have been told through advertising and bad representation that your body is not a body that has value. Yeah, that thought in your brain that says your body is odd was made via the constant stream of images you see that don't look like you. That internalized oppression could start making itself known in the form of physical self-critique—remember to be critical of its existence in your brain. When you expose yourself to yourself, you tell your brain that your beautiful body is 100 percent normal. Repeat, repeat, repeat.

10| EMBRACE CHANGE. Things change, people change, bodies change, the world changes. It's inevitable. Accepting change can be difficult because it really hits on our need for control—maybe this is something you noticed in the emotional triggers exercise. The thing is, bucking against change is like fighting a current. Change is going to happen, but it might be rough and snag a few rocks as it flows. Flow with the stream, and look inward to yourself to find (emotionally mature) ways to feel comfortable within that chaos. If you're struggling with your self-esteem amid the change, then consider therapy. There is no shame in asking for help when you need it.

STOP! IN THE NAME OF LOVING YOURSELF! Not only do we need to hear that we are good from others, but we also need to hear it from ourselves, from within! Feelings around nudity and sexiness are significantly more mental than they are physical. Don't believe me? Next time you have a great day, write down how you feel about your body. Then do the same when you have a bad day. The difference will be drastic. That's because our self-perception comes from our mental attitude and not the physicality of our bodies. Want to change the way you see yourself? Prioritize your mental health first:

- Fill your social feed with people who look like you!

- Add in people who don't look like you and come from different backgrounds!

- Be as naked as you can for as long as you can.

- Get to know your body more through masturbation! For folks who experience physical dysphoria, focus on the parts of your body you are comfortable with: Try applying your favorite lotion to those areas or softly caressing yourself. Make it a game to discover pleasurable sensations in unexpected areas.

- Enjoy a good night's sleep.

- Surround yourself with people who are jazzed to see you.

The Inner Saboteur

Let me introduce you to someone you will have to deal with for your entire life: The Inner Saboteur (or the inner critic, as it is called in psychology) is that little voice inside your head that tells you you're not good enough, smart enough, *blank* enough for the world. It's that voice that comes out on bad days, the voice that tells you you're worthless. The Inner Saboteur is part of your psyche, and it can hijack your conscious mind when you feel uncomfortable. Its function is to protect you by reminding you that the world is a scary, dangerous place where you need to avoid mistakes. But the Inner Saboteur isn't great at thinking critically, which stops you from growing when it tries to guard you from risk.

As I worked on my own body image and self-confidence, my Inner Saboteur would show up when things got hard to tell me that I didn't deserve to love myself or connect with my body. I started using various tactics to manage my Inner Saboteur, so that it couldn't get the best of me. One of the best things you can do for yourself on this journey to self-love and self-acceptance is to learn to quiet that inner critic.

HOW TO MANAGE THE INNER SABOTEUR

The truth is, you're never going to completely get rid of that voice. Experience will make it easier to manage, and time will mellow it, but it will always be there. So instead of trying to fight that voice off, we can learn how to master it.

1| NAME YOUR INNER SABOTEUR. I see mine as this overgrown, child-adult dinosaur named Saboteurus rex.

2| WHEN YOU HEAR YOUR INNER SABOTEUR PUT YOU DOWN, RESPOND WITH: "Thank you for contributing. We will table this discussion for later."

3| INVOKE A ROUTINE—a self-care routine, an anger management routine, a skin-care routine—any routine will do. Routines are calming, and their familiarity helps us ignore the Inner Saboteur and run on autopilot when we're feeling less than.

4| PLEASURE YOURSELF. This can be sexual or otherwise. Your Inner Saboteur might tell you that doing good things for yourself is indulgent, but these are the small moments in life that make it all worth it!

5| SET UP BOUNDARIES. Give your Inner Saboteur times it can and cannot come out. Do we want it to come out? Probably not. But sometimes we just need to cry and feel all of our feelings so we can get back to critically thinking about what we need.

COMPLIMENT YOURSELF

Here's a challenge I think you're up for: Stand naked in front of a mirror and say 10 nice things about yourself that aren't physical. It's just you, your body, and compliments galore! Ready? Go!

Date Accomplished: _____

Rephrasing Phrases

The common thread in my story—my life, my career, and pretty much everything I do—comes back to my body size and weight. I've spent so much time thinking that my weight was the thing holding me back, when in reality it is and always has been the thing that makes me passionate and caring and active in this life. Loving ourselves and embracing who we are should be a human right, but we have been trained to hate our bodies in order to be manipulated by the latest, greatest, next idea in beauty standards. And because of this, we tell ourselves things that are deeply harmful to our bodies, our brains, and possibly the people around us. Let's get rephrasing.

"I FEEL FAT" (TO MEAN YOU'RE FULL OR NO LONGER HUNGRY).

Fat is not a feeling, but rather a reclamation of identity by fat-identified folks. This phrase should be reconsidered, as it diminishes people's experience. You can say:

"I feel full."

"I feel like I honored my hunger."

If someone offers you food, simply say, *"I am good right now. No thank you!"*

"YOU LOOK AMAZING. HAVE YOU LOST WEIGHT?"

Let's all try to stop associating weight loss with a better quality of life. You can say:

"I love your dress."

"You look happy today."

"I ALREADY ATE DESSERT THIS WEEK. NO MORE FOR ME."

Restriction is really interesting because the moment you take something away, the harder it is to ignore that craving. Instead of limiting your intake of sweets, reframe this thought in a more neutral way. You can say:

"There are days where I'm going to want more sweets than other days."

"I'm going to listen to how my body feels this week."

"Food is neutral, not good or bad."

DEVELOPING BOUNDARIES

We know our story, we are cultivating self-worth, we are embracing ourselves. Next up: boundaries. That is, what we will and won't do. Chances are, we already have some boundaries in place.

If we really think about it, there are so many ways in which our body boundaries are crossed all the time. Parents tell children to hug adults when they don't want to, white people literally touch Black people's hair (we must stop this), the media finds it perfectly OK to make comments about other people's bodies and appearances, we force people to eat (clean your plate!) or not eat (you're going to order that?), and men in power routinely get away with touching women's bodies, as we've seen over and over (hello #MeToo). It's really terrifying and unbelievable.

Look, the world is a scary, unpredictable place with nuance and accidents, but also with premeditated, problematic issues. We can't protect ourselves from everything. But what we can do is establish strong boundaries for ourselves in terms of what we will or won't do. Not only is this a great personal growth opportunity to come face-to-face with our internal wants and needs, but it also allows us to practice being clear with others who have access to our bodies and brains.

PERSONAL BOUNDARIES: MOVING THROUGH THE YESES AND NOS
Boundaries are there to keep us mentally and emotionally safe, and expressing those boundaries to ourselves, friends, and lovers is a form of self-love and self-care. What are some of your day-to-day "HARD nos"? Feel free to write them in the book or in a notebook. See mine:

- Fatphobic conversations or comments—I will not engage.
- Heels—Nah.

- Lateness—I can't be late, and I am very clear with friends, coworkers, family, and peers about my feelings on lateness.

- Men who try to explain things to me that I'm an expert on. "The body-positive movement is . . ." should never come out of your mouth near me.

Boundaries in Relationships

A boundary is also an invisible barrier between you and other people that you will not approach or cross beyond. It is not what people are allowed to do, but rather how you react to someone else's behavior. Spending time developing your interpersonal boundaries gives you an internal sense of where your feelings of safety start and stop.

HEALTHY BOUNDARIES

- Trusting appropriately

- Maintaining personal values despite others' opinions

- Saying no to things you don't want: food, touch, affection, gifts, sex

- Asking a person before touching them

- Knowing who you are and what you want

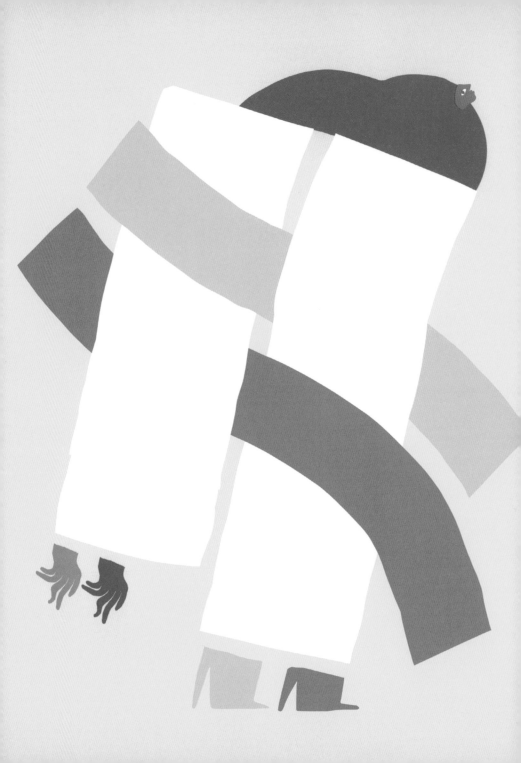

UNHEALTHY BOUNDARIES (OR SIGNS OF NONEXISTENT BOUNDARIES)

- Falling in love at the first sign of affection

- Trusting no one . . . or trusting everyone

- Accepting food, touch, gifts, or sex that you don't want

- Touching another person without their expressed consent (see chapter 5 for more on consent)

- Letting others disrespect your identities or deny (gaslight) your experiences

- Allowing others to invade your boundaries without standing up for yourself

Let's Practice Boundary Setting

Following are a few common scenarios in life and dating that require us to make a decision on behalf of ourselves. We want to get our boundaries in our bones so we feel more than confident if and when we need to whip one out during our sexual and self-love journey. Choose one of the following options or write in your own boundary-applying phrase. Then say it confidently 5 times in front of a mirror!

SCENARIO 1: *Your coworker wants you to stay and have one more drink, but you don't want to. No matter the reason. You don't want to. After some pushing on their part, you can say:*

"I really appreciate the offer, but I'm going to go home and rest for tomorrow."

"No thank you. I'll see you on Monday!"

"You have fun."

"Hey hey, I said no."

SCENARIO 2: *Your date is making a lot of sexual innuendos and you're like, I get it, but I'm not interested in being sexual today or with this date. You can say:*

"Love the confidence, but you're playing to the wrong audience."

"What are your intentions here? I'm trying to enjoy the night, but I'm feeling a little uncomfortable that you keep bringing up _____."

"Hey! I'm having fun! Let's leave the sex talk for another time when I consent to it."

"I'm not sure where you got that this was a sex-only or sex-talk date, but I don't think I gave any indication of that."

"I'm not going to have sex tonight/today."

SCENARIO 3: *You're in the middle of sex and your sexual partner does something or says something that you find to be really offensive or uncomfortable. You can say:*

"Stop. I don't like that."

"One second. That is not something I enjoy. Let's continue doing the other thing we were doing, and we can chat later about some sexual boundaries."

"(Safe word)." (More on safe words on page 205!)

"Oooh . . . can you say/do something else? That word/action doesn't make me feel great."

> *Stop being nice to people who are garbage and don't respect your boundaries.*

Kindness is great. We should all strive to be loving and empathetic with the people in our lives. But. But. But. The biggest but (and not the good kind of butt): Kindness can also allow wrongful behavior to come off as acceptable, or it can be misinterpreted as a "go-ahead" to take things a step further.

Let me be crystal clear here: Kindness isn't an excuse for sexual misconduct. Kindness isn't a green light for the other party to push further. Kindness doesn't mean "you're asking for it."

We fear that if we aren't kind, then we will somehow lose some moral ground or be considered fussy, hard to work with, unhelpful . . . all things we have told self-identifying women to never ever be, because it isn't "ladylike" or polite. Well, fuck that. If someone even goes near your boundary, you have the right to make sure the sternness in your voice is coming across as clear as day. It sends a message:

No, this isn't OK.
No, you shouldn't do this again.
No, I'm uninterested.
No, this is not professional.
No, you're garbage.

PEOPLE-PLEASER SYNDROME A person who cares more about others' perception of them than their own is suffering from People-Pleaser Syndrome. They act compliant, agreeable, and passive in every situation so as not to rock the boat. Any gender can experience People-Pleaser Syndrome. Biological predisposition, cultural beliefs, familial history, trauma, and social currency all contribute to this syndrome. To remedy People-Pleaser Syndrome:

- Develop boundaries.

- Practice saying no.

- Say no in real-world scenarios.

- Prioritize the things you care about.

- Ask yourself how you benefit first in every scenario.

- If your mental health and/or experiences with trauma are making it hard for you to have boundaries, consider getting support from a trauma-informed therapist.

WHAT ARE YOUR BODY BOUNDARIES RIGHT NOW?

Things change, people change. What we feel today might be different from what we feel tomorrow. But today, my dear reader, we are focusing on our boundaries. Right here, right now.

Draw a map of your body. Get creative! Use markers, pens, glitter, crayons, collage. Make it as YOU as you want!

Create a key for your map. In a moment, you will be circling different sections of the body in a specific color. That color will represent a type of touch you'd like or not like to receive. Red means no touching whatsoever, green means touch by a lover, orange means touch by a friend, yellow means touch by a family member, and purple means touch by an acquaintance.

Begin circling (or adding a star) to the areas you do and don't want to be touched using the represented colors. For example, in red, I'd like you to circle where you don't want to be touched no matter the circumstance. Write down any specific types of touch you don't want. If you'd like, write down why.

Continue to circle (or star) with each color, making notes as you continue, so that you feel solid in the physical boundaries of your body.

Having a physical map in your possession will help mentally solidify your boundaries and serve as a reminder of who you are and what you want.

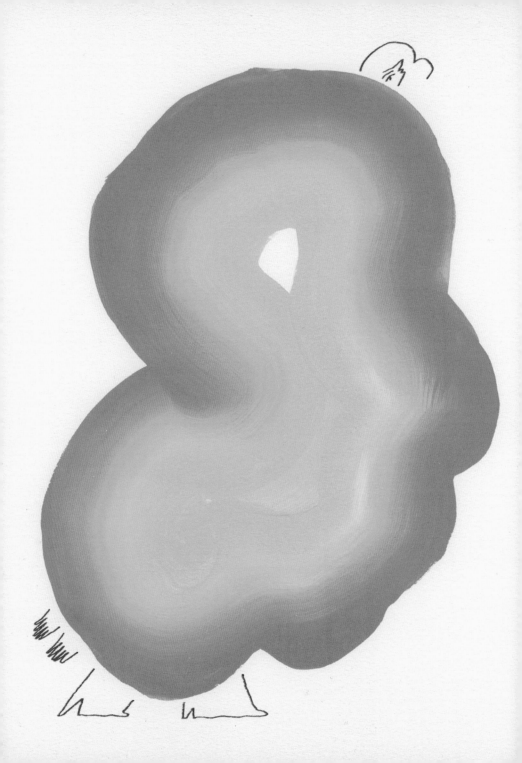

2

How to

Love

Yourself

First

Imagine your ideal date. Maybe there is an activity. Maybe you get something to eat. You wink at yourself every time you pass a mirror because you're looking so good.

The sexual tension is unparalleled. All your needs are met and none of your boundaries are crossed. The whole night is magical, and you know you deserve the best of what this night has to offer. Amazing, right? Guess what. You can have this right now.

DATE YOURSELF

In this chapter, we're not going to worry about other people for a bit and just concentrate on ourselves. When we date other people, we try to put our best foot forward, we give it our all, and we listen to their backstory, but sometimes we forget about our own. We concern ourselves over whether they like iced coffee with or without almond milk. Because we care.

But right now, it's time to care about yourself, because you deserve it.

Yes, you! You, the person looking to find more ways to connect with yourself. You, the person looking to find more meaningful relationships with others. You, the person who wants (and deserves) a hot sex life at no expense to your emotional well-being. You're at the center of this, and taking some time to date yourself is an essential step to discovering what you like, dislike, and don't need.

When you know who you are, you're more likely to make better, more considered decisions in life and in the bedroom. Remember chapter 1? Your pleasure isn't just physical; it's mental and emotional too. Taking the time to understand ourselves mentally will make the physicality of hot sex that much hotter. So that's where we have to start. Feel me?

WHAT I MEAN WHEN I SAY "DATE YOURSELF"

The Yeses

- Spending time getting to know who you are

- Exploring your comfort (and discomfort) zones

- Asking yourself difficult questions

- Going on an actual date with yourself

- Nourishing your body with food that it loves

The Nos

- Saying "fuck it" and doing anything you want

- Running up a credit card bill

- Making irrational decisions

- Calling exes to say, "I don't need you, bitch!" (Though, if you need to scream that into a pillow, I'm not going to stop you.)

We've been fed the idea that in order to be happy and fulfilled, we need to be in constant search for The One. That in order to experience true pleasure, someone has to come and give it to us. That in order to really love our body, we need to be admired by others and gain as many likes from social media as possible.

Well, what if I told you The One was you all along?

THE POWER OF BEING WITH YOU

We have been taught that our value comes from other people's acceptance of us.

We see this in pop culture and the sex industry and the idea that we need to have sex or be sexual in order to gain affection. We see this in body image and diet culture, which have made us believe that in order to be considered hot, we need to have a certain body type. We see this in the institution of marriage and the belief that one person is supposed to be the be-all and end-all of our existence, even if respect is not there.

The reality is that you have every single thing you need inside of you to feel valued. Dating yourself and learning to be with yourself allows you to be more connected to who you are—self-love, body acceptance, and great sex will follow.

THE BEST REASONS TO BE WITH YOURSELF

Choosing to be on your own for a while lets you prioritize yourself and thus:

· Develop hobbies and interests that are important to you.

· Deepen your own sexual exploration and boundaries (more on this in chapter 3).

· Be mindful about what you want and need.

· Have purchasing power over what you want and need without relying on anyone else.

· Live by your time, your energy, your schedule.

· Have the gift of answering to no one (except yourself).

· Control your own time to complete (or not complete) any projects you have in mind.

There is a lot of power in being alone. It allows us to really connect with who we are and what we want. When left to our own devices, our bodies and brains naturally gravitate toward what we inherently care about (intuition is wild). Alone time also provides the calm we need to find our clarity. But, of course, not everyone loves alone time. In fact, if I'm being honest, reader, I feared being alone for quite some time. I feared loneliness. I still do on occasion. And while the most isolating time of my life (during the COVID-19 pandemic) was also a time where I became more connected to my own interests, it was still incredibly difficult. Maybe you can relate?

Being alone and feeling lonely are two different experiences. Loneliness is the absence of connection. While we're not going to feel 100 percent connected all the time, it's worth noting when we feel disconnected or lonely, and why, so we know how to regain that connection. Following are a few different types of loneliness and tips on how to deal when the anxiety of being alone or lonely begins to spike.

- PHYSICAL LONELINESS: Being alone in your home, apartment, or some other space. Physical loneliness can be isolating and make you question who you are and what you deserve. To combat physical loneliness, try taking a walk, calling a friend, visiting a museum, taking yourself out on a date, and experiencing the world outside of yourself.

- EMOTIONAL LONELINESS: Feeling alone in your feelings, as if no one understands you or you can't share your true emotions. To combat emotional loneliness, try journaling, reading a book, donating, or volunteering, so that you're acting in service to others rather than ruminating in your inner world and dwelling on your feelings.

- ROMANTIC LONELINESS: Not having a partner. I can't remember a moment in my life when I wasn't fed the narrative that if I wasn't married, engaged, or in a loving, committed (read: monogamous) relationship, then I was basically damaged goods. The vast majority of movies and TV shows—consider the entire Disney canon, the Bridget Jones franchise, or every rom-com ever—are dedicated to the idea that in order to be a valued human, another human needs to accept you and grant you that value. To combat romantic loneliness, try having special nights just for you, creating a passion project that has no monetary incentive, or spending time outlining your goals. Be there for yourself more than wanting someone else to be there for you.

On Being Alone At thirty-one, I uprooted my life and moved into a studio apartment. I was under the impression that I needed to do so in order to feel like an adult. Before the move, I was living with roommates and feeling like it wasn't for me anymore. Not because I had bad roommates, but because I had thought I would be (or should be) more independent at that point in my life. From the moment I made my decision all the way to the day before I moved out of my studio apartment (literally twenty-nine days), I tried to understand why I would do something that I clearly wasn't ready for.

The answer: I didn't listen to myself or my needs, nor did I stop to understand why I wanted to be in my own place. Through a lot of consideration, therapy, and analysis of the situation, I realized that I was unhappy and unable to move forward in my career at the time, and that insecurity made me feel like I needed to make a larger adult decision.

I learned a lot about myself from that experience. First and foremost, I learned that I am uncomfortable with how others perceive my adulthood. This hidden discomfort was running around my brain like a toddler with a knife just waiting to cause damage when unearthed.

I'm not saying you should make a big life decision in order to learn big life lessons. I'm saying that the next time you feel uncomfortable being alone, ask yourself why. Is it because it's scary? Is it because you feel unprepared? Is it because you have to be with your own thoughts? Those answers will help inform your decision-making and determine your readiness for the next step in your life, whether that's moving into your own apartment, taking a solo vacation, entering into a new relationship, or anything else.

If you're having a hard time with loneliness, that's totally OK. If you find yourself in an alone position and can't enjoy it without negative thoughts getting in the way, consider what you can do to combat those feelings at their root rather than jumping into something that might temporarily ease the loneliness but that isn't healthy in the long run.

My dearest reader, I would love nothing more than for you to enjoy your own company. We fill our days and brains with all kinds of distractions that get in the way of what we actually want and need. Ignoring those personal prompts allows us to be easily swayed, prioritize others over our own well-being, and make decisions that are truly not in our best interest. It isn't always easy to listen to what YOU have to say—goodness knows we all have some version of imposter syndrome inside of us. But it's important to be able to enjoy being alone and to find value in your independence.

Now that we're committed to exploring our alone time, let's make the most of it by identifying and enjoying our pleasures.

SOLO DATES

Ah, yes, yes, yes—the solo date. The time in which you are in control of what you do, where you go, and how the night will end. A freewheeling night where you are your own date and the world is your big, wide-open oyster!

Why go on a solo date? Well, because it's fun, you get to pick the itinerary, and it's an excellent way to show yourself how you like and deserve to be treated by yourself and by other people. Get this: Our brain responds to patterns!

WHAT WOULD YOU CONSIDER THE PERFECT DAY?

For real. If you were to lay out for me—nay, for yourself—your perfect day, what would it be? The best part about dating yourself and being a self-considered babe is that you get to decide what a perfect day looks like for you, and then make it happen (to the best of your ability, of course). There is such power in treating yourself with respect and love, especially considering that we all have an inner saboteur that would love nothing better than to replay every single uncomfortable, sad, embarrassing moment over and over until we believe it. The more we take care of ourselves, the easier it is to find that self-love—and through that, it's easy to see how beautiful our bodies actually are. So now, what is your ideal date? Write it down in this book or in a preferred notebook so you can recall it (and act upon it!) on your next free day.

PROMPT: What does your perfect day look like? (Feel free to describe both a realistic and an unrealistic version, if you'd like.)

SET UP THE PERFECT SOLO DATE

Above all else, you come first. Your happiness comes first. And what is a better way to show that for yourself than to have a night (or morning) that is completely dedicated to you? Here are a few ideas:

- Create an elaborate meal for yourself.

- People watch at a local cafe or wine bar.

- Go to a show or an outdoor event by yourself.

- Take a long walk.

- Go to the movies! Or recreate the experience at home.

- Walk around a museum . . . and maybe bring a sketchbook!

- Go to a luxurious dinner or spa.

- Book a hotel room for a night!

- Listen to audio erotica while drinking wine at a local cafe.

- Spend the whole night nude taking hot photos of yourself.

HOW TO TAKE A NUDE

The coolest part of dating yourself is that you can explore your own carnal needs without the pressure of another person, and that can be really fun if you have access to a camera or a smartphone. Nudes, and especially nude selfies, are high art, an ode to the self, a memento that you actually exist. They're an excellent reminder of just how hot you really are—especially when you're having a bad day. They are for you to have or share as you see fit. (I'd like to take this moment to remind you that I'd love for us to live in a perfect world with perfect people, but sadly this is not the case. Leaked nudes are nonconsensual breaches by horrible people—that's it. Take extra care here.)

- First, remind yourself that your naked body is glorious. It deserves to be photographed.

- Use natural lighting throughout the space, and avoid overhead light at all costs.

- Practice your poses—it's harder than it looks!

- Set up your camera—or camera phone—so the lens is looking straight at you. (Use a chair or books to prop it up if needed.) Or try something unique by placing the camera at a low angle for you to hover over it. Yes, maybe you see a double chin . . . but who cares? This is a major power position!

- Add props or a mirror for a little depth.

- Stretch and move before you take the photos—feel good in your body.

- Play a little empowering or sexy music to make this moment extra fun!

- Experiment with different back-drops, using scarves, at-home objects, or bedding to create a unique environment. Try out different kinds of makeup looks, hairstyles, or other ways of adjust-ing your appearance. You could even follow a makeup tutorial that teaches camera makeup (i.e., makeup that will show up best on camera).

- If you prefer to have part of your body obscured because of dysphoria (or artistic reasons), try wrapping scarves around that part of your body, use your hands or other body parts to cover that part of yourself, or even wear lingerie that partially covers your body and helps you feel powerful and sexy.

- Take the photos using the timed-release setting. Or better yet, take one continuous video and pause/screenshot the frames you like!

- Preview with kindness. Your body is your body is your body.

Soloing as a Self-Esteem Builder

For a super fun, self-esteem-building solo date (a two-for-one!), why not try something a little outside your comfort zone?

Of course, when doing something for the first time, you're going to be scared! Your brain will travel to the worst possible scenario, providing all the reasons why you shouldn't be doing what you're doing. You might psyche yourself out of the experience because of a fear of failing. Let me tell you a secret: This feeling happens to everyone. Yes, everyone. Even Zac Efron. Even your mom. Even me—hell, it happens to me every time I go to a workout class by myself (I get nervous and self-conscious about people judging me!). But showing yourself you can do what you want on your own helps build your self-esteem. Is some of it going to be within the realm of emotionally scary? Yes, possibly. But this is why we need to try it so we can feel empowered by that accomplishment!

LATEST SOLO DATES I TOOK MYSELF ON . . . AND THEIR SCORES

1| TOOK A DANCE CLASS: Let me tell you . . . the whole thing was painful. I'm all for movement and stretching and dancing, but dear goodness, this was not for me. 3/10

2| BAKED CROISSANTS: It took forever and they definitely didn't look even close to Parisian, but they were so tasty! 10/10

3| WORE ORANGE WHILE TAKING A WALK THROUGH THE CITY: I'm a New Yorker forever with a noir-style closet to match. But adding bright-colored clothes to my otherwise all-black theme brings me little bits of joy. 7/10

4| STRETCHED IN THE MORNING: I always thought stretches were for elite athletes. . . . Well, consider me a gold medalist because, dang, morning stretches are the best thing to ever happen to my life, especially because I walk a lot! 8/10

5| HAD A PASTA NIGHT IN SOHO: Just me, my red wine, penne, and a pile of bread. People walked by, looked in my direction, and kept walking. Sure, it made me self-conscious, but it was so worth it. It was a night just for me and it was exactly what I needed. 10/10

NAME YOUR PLEASURES

The first step in dating yourself is to declare it. You need to make this relationship official! There is so much to be said for expressing your goals out loud. Not only do you hear it, but the universe also hears it, and you immediately put some positive intentions out into the world.

If you will indulge me (and yourself) for a second, I'd love for you to take a moment for yourself and say this phrase. You may even want to look at your glowing self in a mirror when you say it (up to you!).

Oh, hey! You are so smart and so fine. I can't wait to get to know you more, _____(fill in your name). Let's learn more about you, be kind in whatever we discover, and remember that we get to live this one life the way we want to, ya hot peach!

Declaration, done! Congrats, you're now officially dating yourself! No big hoopla here. Simply a verbal commitment to getting to know yourself a little deeper over the course of this chapter, this book, and your life outside of these pages.

Dear Reader, No matter where you were emotionally when you picked up this book, how much confidence you had or have, or how much you've already worked on yourself, there is always room for improvement. There will never be a day where everything is suddenly fine—life isn't that simple. Of course, feel free to date or keep dating others as you learn to date yourself. Dating yourself is simply an opportunity to learn more about yourself and love yourself for who you are. *Capisce?*

The second step in dating yourself is to name your pleasures. Pleasures, much like self-care, are a means to creating a life that we love to live. Pleasures have just as much to do with sexual needs and wants as they do with tangible, non-sexy objects or feelings that we covet. They are the little things that don't cost much or don't cost anything at all that make our days, months, and years so much more satisfying. They're tiny moments and things that make us feel at ease. They are the bread crumbs that form a path back to who we are and what we love. Not only are pleasures wildly fun, but they also come in handy when we're not feeling like ourselves or need some respite.

WHAT WOULD BE CONSIDERED A PLEASURE?

A pleasure can be anything as long as it makes you feel good. Other people be damned, this is about you! A pleasure could be a fruit that is cut up in a certain way. It could be quiet time. It could be a full-on sexual fantasy. It could even be spending a whole day inside writing while wearing leopard-print spandex (not that I'm speaking from personal experience or anything . . .).

AREN'T PLEASURES EXTRAVAGANT?

The difference between pleasures and extravagant indulgences is that the latter are an escape from the world. They don't take into account any long-term ramifications on our

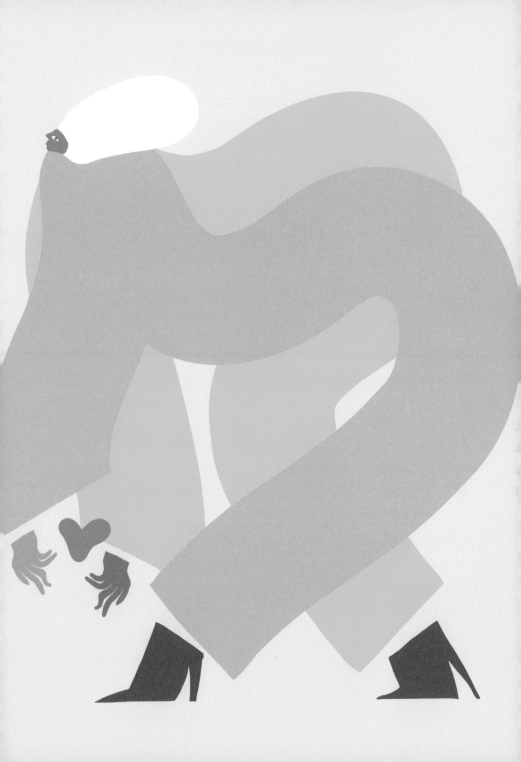

physical and emotional well-being. Pleasures enhance the life we are building; they are not an escape. If a pleasure could be a square of premium dark chocolate, then an extravagance could be a massive box of processed chocolate candy (I have enjoyed both). Really consider this in all the things you do, reader. Is the thing in front of you allowing you to be present in life or escape from it?

HOW DO I FIND MY PLEASURES?

What interests you? What things make you incredibly happy? They can be something as simple as lemon-ginger tea before bed. Sometimes you think you like something and then you try it and realize you don't. No big deal! Your pleasures list can evolve and change over time. Much of pleasure seeking is trial and error, and it's a part of getting to know yourself.

WHAT IF I'M SUPPOSED TO LIKE SOMETHING THAT I DON'T LIKE?

Let's take a second to address this. It's so important to remember that just because you were socialized to like something doesn't mean you need to like it, such as being friends with people who make you feel bad about yourself or even hugging a family member who has made you feel uncomfortable. Life is honestly too damn short to not be doing the things you want to do.

HOW TO GET COMFORTABLE WITH LIFE'S PLEASURES

Many of us have been taught not to engage in the things we love and care about for fear they are too indulgent, too independent, too odd. And so, it can be difficult to think about engaging in the things we like. Let's work on getting comfortable with our pleasures.

- Create a running list of the things that give you pleasure in life (see the activity on page 81). When you're having a particularly hard day, it's a nice reminder that you can select from a handful of options that will make the rest of your day that much easier.

- Say them out loud. In the same way you declared your commitment to yourself, declare your commitment to having a pleasurable life.

- Create full rituals around your pleasures. Rituals, or routines, connect us back to who we are. (See page 82 for ideas.)

My Pleasures I hope you enjoy this beautifully eclectic list of my pleasures that tether me back to who I am. Start thinking of your own.

- Lengthwise slices of white peaches

- Really comfortable Adidas slides

- Turning off notifications

- Hot yoga classes that bring out an emotion

- Afternoon sex

- Rose scents (my bathroom smells like a garden)

- Laying my face on a round butt

- Very pretty dead flowers that I don't have to worry about killing

- Listening to a podcast while cooking an elaborate meal

- A perfectly shaped butt plug

- One-on-one friendship time (I'm really bad in group settings)

- A fresh set of acrylic nails

- Hot pink lipstick (even if it makes me look like a depressed Barbie)

- Selfies in new lingerie (I love keeping reminders of when I felt the sexiest)

- Cartoons for adults

- Stationery. I love pens; I love notebooks. To the rulers of the digital sphere, you will not take these away from me no matter how cool your note-taking technology is.

WHAT ARE YOUR PLEASURES?

OK, reader. It's time to write them down. What are the things in your life that give you a little bit of comfort when the world feels nonsensical? Write them in this book or in a notebook or on your phone. Have them, cherish them, be good to them, because these are the things that are going to be good to you when you need it. And even more than that, write down why they matter to you. This list can be revamped any time; it should be ever-changing based on who you are and what you love.

Not sure where to start? That's OK! Here are a few silly, sexy, weird yes-or-no questions to prompt your list.

- Bubble wrap: Yes or no?

- Early riser or night owl?

- Soft fabrics or structured fit?

- Sleeping nude or silky pajamas?

- Rewatching your favorite show or discovering something new?

- Hot showers or bubble baths?

- Mountains or ocean?

- Productive or chill Sundays?

CULTIVATE RITUALS

Rituals ground us. They are a reminder that yes, things will turn back around. Just like our pleasures, our rituals take care of us, embrace us, and serve as a reminder that loving our body and having great sex is something we deserve.

RITUALS ARE ALSO AN IMPORTANT FORM OF SELF-CARE

- Rituals are created based on our decision to feel good!

- Rituals allow us to strive for our personal goals and keep us accountable.

- Rituals teach us to put ourselves first.

- Rituals hold space for us to be truly present.

- Rituals reinforce that we deserve to feel pleasure.

Types of Rituals

You can create your own rituals or ritual categories for self-love. Here are some of my favorites.

SELF-CARE RITUALS connect you back to yourself. A self-care ritual could be journaling, doing a skin-care regimen, getting a haircut, reorganizing your home, sleeping in, or taking care of a plant. This is your time to feel good about yourself and in your surrounding space. For example, sometimes when I'm feeling stressed, I take a long walk through my city to clear my head. My computer is away, my phone is on silent, and all I can do is concentrate on putting one foot in front of the other.

A SELF-CARE TIP: *Spend the entire day in a bathrobe. Take a shower, apply your best sheet masks, have a lovely breakfast, and luxuriate. We are always busy, always on the move, always doing the most. When we give ourselves a little love, our body will thank us, and our mind will start to believe that we don't need to suffer in order to relax.*

SEXUAL RITUALS are the various ways you take care of yourself in your upcoming, current, or future sexual experiences. This could be remembering to carry a condom or lube packets with you, making personal rules around protection for future hook-ups and lovers, or communicating before getting naked with another person. Basically, it's the 1, 2, 3s before les activités sexuelles. For example, I always take a moment to talk about sex when I'm on dates. After I've spent some time with and gotten to know this other person quite well, I'll ask, "Would you be into speaking about sex, boundaries, or general intimacy right now?" If they say no, we put a mental "pin" in it. If they say yes, I make sure they are enthusiastic about the convo before I continue. Sure, it's very hot and definitely a fun way to see what the other person is into, but it also presents me with the opportunity to state my boundaries.

BE BEDSIDE PREPARED: *Take an hour to create a little bedside kit of everything you might need for the best sexual experience— latex, latex-free, or nitrile gloves, condoms, dental dams, lube, batteries, chargers, essential oils, sex toys, you name it. Put it somewhere accessible so you can grab it and go without having to disrupt your flow.*

HEARTBREAK RITUALS are the ways you protect your heart as well as handle heartbreak from others. The heart will love and break and mend and move on and find love again. During that cycle, it's so important to listen to yourself and what you need. If you could give your brokenhearted self some advice from the future you, what would it be? Mine would be: Laura, you have so much value even if you can't see it right now. Go do something you love because you are more than this feeling. Acknowledge it, feel it, but don't let it consume you.

REALLY CRY: *There is no use in bottling all your feelings inside. They will always make their way through your body and out into the open one way or another. So really feel what you're feeling. Write it all down and get it out of your body, if that helps, and process at your own pace.*

ANGER RITUALS are strategies you can use when you go from 0 to 100 on the angry scale. When, say, you get a wild email at work (me) or someone makes you mad. I know myself well enough to know that I need to walk away for a good 10 minutes before I can respond to anyone when I'm pissed off—and sometimes I have to leave it for 72 hours before I let myself have a reaction.

USE THAT ENERGY FOR GOOD: *Instead of replying with "Per my last email . . . ," take a moment and write a list of everything that was great today. It could be as simple as "I really got in there when brushing my teeth" (I would 100 percent write this). Remind yourself of all the good things you did today before dealing with the situation at hand.*

GO-TO RITUALS

- Early morning walks

- Baking every Sunday morning

- Daily sketches in a notebook

- Reading the paper during breakfast

- Telling yourself that you're a bad bitch every morning

(for all of you self-identified bad bitches out there)

- Nightly skin-care routine

- Playing music right before bed

- Foot stretches to keep them limber

Good Nights Lead to Good Mornings

When we take care of ourselves, we see that care reflected across every aspect of our life—and a great night's sleep can lead to more positive decision-making the next day. A nightly self-care ritual grounds us within ourselves, our bodies, and our awareness. So, let's develop one just for you!

- SPEND QUALITY TIME BRUSHING AND FLOSSING YOUR TEETH. Really get in there! Brushing your teeth and taking time to do it is hygienic, it wards off future dental pain, and it teaches you to slow down and be mindful about what you want and need.

- SKIN CARE CAN BE REALLY FUN WHEN YOU GET INTO IT! Pick a brand or a step-by-step process that works best for your skin, and stick with it! Even on late nights when I'm a few too many red wines in (two and I'm destroyed), I will force myself to take off my cat-eye liner and moisturize my skin. If you can get into the habit, not only will your skin feel great, but you will also be more likely to translate that "me first" attitude to other parts of your life.

- PICK UP A GOOD READ. Oh, hey! You're already doing it! Our brain is always on; our eyes are always glued to a screen. Give the screen a rest each night so that your brain can be mentally relaxed when drifting off to sleep.

- FEELING SEXY? Porn is a great option, but have you ever read an erotic novel? Babe, let me tell you . . . get ready to have an amazing solo orgasm. Sexual play can be more than rolling around with a partner. Sex toys can also be a really fun part of a stellar nighttime ritual. Leaving a vibrator or lubricant or condoms by the bed is an excellent reminder that you deserve pleasure (more on this in chapter 4). Orgasms help you sleep, so consider incorporating sexy time with your erotica and/or toys before bed.

HOW TO CURATE YOUR SPACE

Create a sanctuary! If we recharged the way we charge our phones, we'd all be energetic creatures without a grumpy bone in our bodies. But that's not how it works—in fact, we are constantly pushing the limits of our exhaustion. Bedtime is for relaxation and comfort, and it's a great opportunity to make your bedroom the most calming, cool, chill room for the best rest of your life. Colors, scents, and low lighting are all great options.

- **SELF-CARE COLORS:** What's your favorite color? Incorporate it wherever you can—whether that means repainting your bedroom walls or simply adding a few accessories. Your bathroom is a great place to highlight some of your favorite colors. My toothbrush is pink, my hairbrush is pink, my face masks are pink. Pink makes me feel really good and playful, and it helps start and end my day.

- **PERSONAL SCENT:** Find your signature scent—or scents—and use it throughout your space via a candle, a diffuser, or incense. Use it on your body, too, with lotions, perfumes, or bubble bath. You can have different scents for different rooms, different moods, or different times of day. A scent can bring back memories, make you feel sexy, or simply be a reminder of who the heck you are (mine is rose)! Have fun with it!

- **CALMING BEDSHEETS:** Look for dark, soft bedsheets that use natural fibers like eucalyptus or bamboo to help ease you into dreamland.

- **LOW LIGHTING:** We are all glued to our screens. I'm guilty of this! Low lights in the bedroom can create a more serene sleeping experience and make us feel less tired in the morning.

- **SEX TOY STORAGE:** Sex toys are often cumbersome to store. Create a little space in your closet to hang harnesses, collars, and handcuffs so that you can always see what is available—and so you remind yourself that you're a mad sexy being every time you look for a pair of socks!

- **ART, ART, ART:** Give your eyes someplace to rest and enjoy soothing colors or a relaxing scene.

Rituals Can't Solve It All

Sadly, not all of us live in a world where we can wake up, drink $10 celery juice, and start working when we feel like it. Most of us have more than one job and we don't have the luxury or leisure to kick back and let the world present its best self to us. Let's just acknowledge this right now so we can remember that things are difficult. We have been thrown quite the hand and there is no way for all of us to walk to the other side of cultural shifts without feeling overwhelmed by the universal state of affairs. We need to give ourselves some grace and kindness. Perfection doesn't allow us to grow, and growth is messy.

Self-care practices can't solve everything, but creating a foundation of self-love via pleasures, solo dates, and positive rituals will help us navigate whatever the world throws our way.

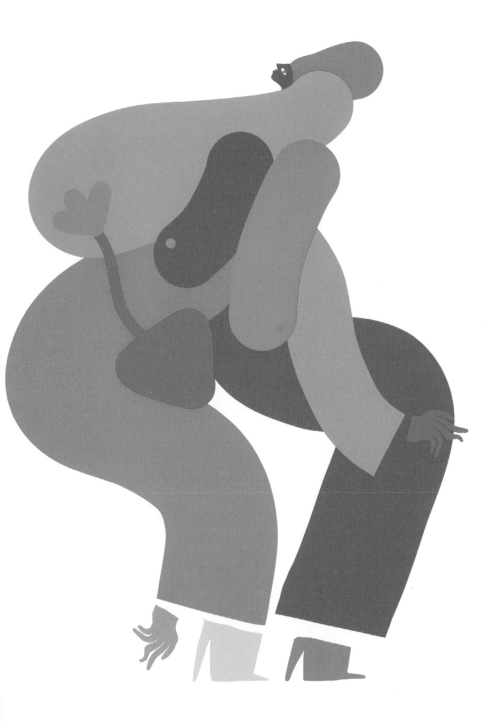

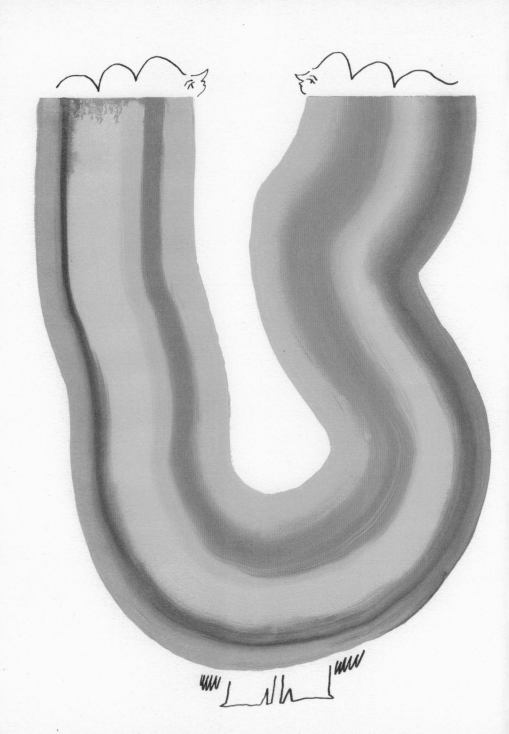

3

Solo

Play

My dearest reader —
Love yourself today,
tomorrow, and every
day after.

To love yourself is to know yourself, and solo play (i.e., mastur-bation) is a singularly perfect way to understand your wants, pleasure points, fantasies, and personal boundaries.

But hey, solo play isn't easy for everyone, and not everyone feels comfortable with it—and that's OK! Whatever your expe-rience is, you're welcome here within these pages.

WHY ENGAGE IN SOLO PLAY?

Solo play is good for you in more ways than one: It brings on relaxation, a kinder temperament, and better sleep, *and* makes you a better communicator when it comes to your sex-ual wants and needs. You literally have all the power in your hands to figure out what you like, don't like, and want more of, and how to get it.

Solo play gives you the agency to have the sex you want to be having. It is a judgment-free zone for you to explore.

So far we have revisited our history, cultivated self-esteem, considered our nonsexual pleasures, and enjoyed our alone time. Now it's time to get into the nitty-gritty of bodily plea-sures: how we can pleasure ourselves, why we should plea-sure ourselves, and how that pleasure can translate to other aspects of our lives. By feeling more connected to our bodies and listening to ourselves instead of external messaging, we can reach the apex of masturbatory freedom. When we touch our bodies, we show ourselves kindness. When we give ourselves pleasure, we let our bodies and brains know we deserve it. It's a full-on cycle of self-love and pleasure!

SETTING BODY AND INTIMACY GOALS

Time to set some goals! We're not talking about #bodygoals or anything that would require you to change your physical appearance. Rather, ask yourself what you want from your body and sex life. Make a list of 5 to 10 goals in your notebook. See mine for some inspiration:

- Walk around naked without slouching.

- Cook myself an elaborate dinner once per week while wearing a robe.

- Focus on touching various parts of my body during masturbation.

- Explore nipple play.

- Sleep naked and alone.

- Be less fearful of my jiggly belly and more accepting of her softness.

- Experience my sexual fantasies in a safe and loving environment.

- Be more mindful of the pleasure I need and communicate that to my partners.

In addition to being the topic of conversation that comes up the most when I'm in the midst of giving sex advice, solo play is the one thing that has consistently allowed me to practice body positivity as fiercely as I do. I spent such a long time hating my body; slowly allowing myself to feel pleasure from it has translated into valuing myself. I cannot recommend it enough.

Let's Take a Second

Pause.

How are we feeling? Are we ready to go forward? Yes? Amazing. Let's do it. Here are 5 reasons to get excited about touching yourself:

1| Gosh, it's going to feel good!

2| Pleasure is transferable; its effects are much greater than just an orgasm.

3| Your confidence will increase even more.

4| There is nothing better than some solo play and a nap. It's the ultimate self-care practice!

5| You deserve it.

So far, we've connected with our hearts and minds. Now, we're going straight for our genitalia. Get your masturbation hat on (I hope you actually have one of those) and let's get into it!

MASTURBATION, HEALTH, AND WELLNESS

The wellness industry has made significant coin telling people to breathe deeply, eat acai bowls, and stretch their way into a clear mind and longer life. I can't deny my appreciation for a loving stretch, a bowl of coconut yogurt, mint-infused water, essential oil baths, and a hot yoga class (yes, I do all of these things). But the wellness industry, while vast, has really left behind masturbation as a tried-and-true, multi-beneficial activity. Why is that? Because we have to talk about people taking their pleasure into their own hands? Because we have to admit that women don't need men to have orgasms? Because sex is taboo, especially any kind of sex that isn't between one man and one woman? Because we'd finally put pleasure on the pedestal it deserves instead of making people fear it?

Wellness is a relative term. Everyone is different. Everyone's body is different and everyone's health makeup is different. Some people are predisposed to having more or less weight on them. Some people snore; some people don't. Some people get itchy when they're about to sneeze (me), and so on and so forth. Therefore, everyone's approach to wellness will be completely different. Some people practice yoga or keep a journal. Some people masturbate. Your wellness practice, and your masturbation practice, should be—no, *needs* to be—tailored to what you like.

> *Sexual pleasure is wellness, and*
> *wellness should be for all.*

THE HEALTH BENEFITS OF MASTURBATING

1| Reduces stress

2| Improves self-esteem and body image

3| Strengthens the pelvic floor

4| Relieves menstrual cramps

5| Reduces muscle tension

6| Promotes better sleep

7| Releases sexual tension

8| Boosts overall mood

You hold the key to what you need and want. It's all about being mindful and listening to yourself. Speaking of mindfulness: That is a word that is tossed around all the time for the sake of wellness, and it happens to be a helpful tool in your wellness and masturbation adventure.

Mindfulness: To be conscious or aware of your actions and the actions around you.

How to Practice Mindfulness

I'm going to tell you right now . . . this is harder than it sounds. Sure, you can find ways to take a breath before every decision or emotional reaction, but the brain is hard to control (remember that Inner Saboteur?). Being mindful takes a lot of practice, forgiveness, and patience, but ultimately it will allow for more clarity around what you need and want.

- Mindfulness allows us to be more open to what turns us on.

- Mindfulness can focus our efforts toward an incredible orgasm.

- Mindfulness keeps us connected to our body.

- Mindfulness allows us to make decisions about what our body likes and dislikes.

Do you see the mind-body-pleasure connection yet? Mindfulness keeps you in the moment and has a direct impact on pleasure. Here are some tips on cultivating mindfulness in your everyday life.

*AN IMPORTANT NOTE, BEFORE WE DIVE IN Breathwork and meditation can make people with PTSD feel more anxious, hyperaroused, or dysregulated. There are many different approaches to breathwork, meditation, and mindfulness, and you should feel encouraged to find an alternate practice that works for you! Seek the help of trauma-informed mental health practitioners to determine your best approach.

- WORK ON BRINGING YOUR MIND BACK TO YOURSELF. This can be done with small steps. When you're hungry or tired, or you want to buy a dress you were served through an Instagram ad, take a moment. Ask yourself what you really want. Do you need to be rushing into this action?

- PAY ATTENTION TO YOUR BREATHING. It's kind of amazing that we all do this thing over and over every day without realizing that it's happening. Breathwork can be a great way to slow down and be more mindful. Try this easy practice: Take a deep breath in for 4 counts, hold for 4 counts, and release for 4 counts.

- READ. READ. READ. Well, you're doing it right now. Reading helps you focus and stay connected to the things at hand.

- MEDITATE! Meditation might seem like an extra 10 to 20 minutes to carve into your already busy day, but it can be a great way to gain perspective and calm your mind.

- TAKE A MINDFUL MOMENT WHEN YOU WAKE UP. Sure, it's super easy to wake up and scroll through your emails and notifications the moment your eyes open. There is something to be said for separating yourself from the things you want to do and the things you have to do right when the day starts. Go for a walk, make yourself some tea, or consider one of your pleasures before jumping into what others need.

Mindfulness is a great way to practice sexual and intimate communication with yourself, your body, and your partner(s).

By creating the mental space to listen to your body's wants and needs, you'll be more apt to identify and address bodily signals of physical and emotional pleasure or pain, and thus have the masturbation session or partnered sex that you want to be having. I know, it's a little self-helpy to consider how the brain and the body connect with each other, but it does work. Think of it this way: You want that earth-shattering orgasm? Listen to yourself.

LET'S WORK OUR PC MUSCLES

PC muscles—a.k.a. pelvic floor muscles, a.k.a. pubococcygeus muscles—are an incredibly important part of our genitalia. No lie . . . it's how we all don't piss ourselves constantly. Think of the PC muscles like a hammock that holds all our reproductive organs and our bladder. Sometimes, we need to reinforce the hammock with some strength training, a.k.a. Kegel exercises.

BUT WHAT ARE WE TRAINING FOR?

Stronger PC muscles:

- Help get rid of lower back pain.
- Help manage painful urination.
- Result in stronger, more controlled orgasms!
- Prevent leakage of all sorts.

HOW TO

Sit in a relaxed position and work on the technique. Begin by tightening your PC muscles—the same muscles you use when you are trying not to pee! Clench and hold for 3 counts. Then rest for 5 counts. Do this for a minute. It's really fun if you pick a particularly boring meeting and do a "workout."

- Extend the time. Gradually increase the length of contractions and relaxations. Work your way up to 10-second contractions and 5-second relaxations.

- Aim high. Try to do at least 30 to 40 Kegels every day. Distributing them throughout the day is better than doing them all at once.

- Diversify. Practice short, 2- to 3-second contractions and releases as well as longer ones.

NOTE: If you find the relaxation stage of this exercise a lot harder than the tightening stage, try speaking to your doctor about being referred to a pelvic floor physical therapist.

HOW SHAME HOLDS US BACK, AND THE ROLE OF SOLO PLAY

Shame, shame, shame, shame.

There is a reason Cersei was forced to walk naked through the streets of the Westeros capital in front of all the townspeople—so that she felt shame over her lusty actions and sins of the flesh, according to the religious powers in the *Game of Thrones* world. (Who knew there would be GoT spoilers in this book?)

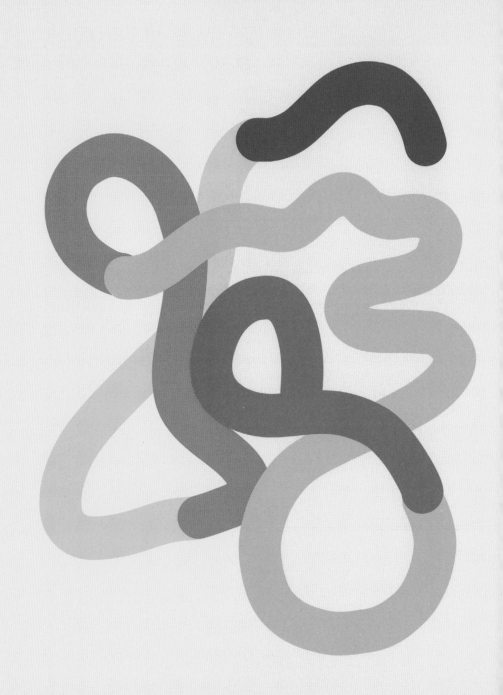

Shame is a weird shape-shifting emotion that can be so much deeper than guilt or embarrassment. It can lower our confidence, build feelings of unworthiness, create a distance between us and others, and make it really difficult to connect to what we love. It can also make it really difficult to be open and honest about what we need—in life, let alone in the bedroom.

We must talk about shame, as it is deeply rooted in how we've been taught to exist in our bodies and experience sexual pleasure. We're taught this at a young age. Puberty can cause feelings of embarrassment when someone other than yourself sees how your body is changing: by having a wet dream, hard nipples, or body hair; by getting your first bra, your period, or a boner in class. The entirety of adolescence is a lot and, unfortunately, many of us were made to feel an intense amount of shame surrounding it. And while it's an emotion, shame can have physical effects on our bodies, as well, including fatigue, chronic pain, and sexual dissatisfaction.

Shame is supremely unfortunate for both your body and your mind.

So, How Do We Get Rid of Shame?

Because shame is inherently about what we think is bad about ourselves, we need to understand where that comes from. In chapter 1, we spoke about our story: where we come from and what led us to who we are today. Now we need to acknowledge that story so we can lower the volume on the shame monster living inside our heads, move forward with our lives, and enjoy sex and pleasure.

1| IDENTIFY: Mentally bookmark the key events from the past that built this shame. This will help get to the root of why you feel a certain way.

2| VARIABLES: Are there other variables to this shame feeling? Are there shame patterns or people in your life who constantly make you feel shame?

3| FIND YOUR CENTER: Take a deep breath, count backward from 10, and take comfort in the fact that shame is an unpleasant emotion but not something that gets to define you.

4| REWORK: Can these moments, patterns, and people be cast in a new light and thought of as a learning opportunity instead of a failure?

I encourage you to consider therapy when processing your relationship with shame. Internalized oppression and shame are deeply connected. For example, LGBTQIA people may internalize societal messaging about their identities and this can lead to feelings of shame about gender, sex, romantic partners, and sexual orientations. I know it's a lot to unpack, but it can lead to a more positive relationship with yourself and others, babes.

THE 90/10 RULE In order to, literally, fuck yourself, you need to mentally unfuck yourself. Ninety percent of sex and masturbation is mental. That means no recounting your to-do list in your head, no worrying about cellulite, and no wondering whether your partner finds you attractive if you arch your back a little higher. This also means navigating your way through shame and coming out on the other side with more self-esteem and a shame-free mentality.

To Deserve or Not to Deserve

Shame is a tricky, prickly little thing that makes you think that you don't deserve anything . . . especially pleasure. And this kind of thinking makes it really difficult to pleasure yourself, to ask for what you want, and to be mindful when a sexual or pleasurable situation isn't up to par.

Pleasure tends to exist in a space in our brains that only opens up when we feel we deserve it, or when we've done XYZ things in order to get to a moment where we can actually enjoy ourselves. I do this . . . I get it. In fact, I tell myself I need to write four emails before I can look at fun things on the internet (memes, cats, rescue pit bull videos that I cry over). But let me just say this: If you deserve to treat yourself to an iced chai latte or a yoga class, which the wellness industry has told us we do, then you deserve to masturbate. It's the same thing, except that masturbation and all versions of sexual pleasure are deeply tied to morality.

Shame, Body Parts, and Common Myths

I think about body parts a lot: the way we interact with them, the way we speak about them, the way we treat them. As someone whose breasts literally walk into a room before I do, I'm hyperaware of how we fetishize and devalue genitalia and body parts.

I was one of those *lucky* students who went through abstinence-only education where an outside instructor came into my classroom and literally passed around a piece of tape to prove that the tape isn't sticky after being used over and over—comparing a vagina to a piece of fucking Scotch tape. After that, the phrase "throwing a hot dog down a hallway" became part of school—a phrase used to shame girls for showing any kind of affection. This kind of thing sticks with us and affects our future relationship to sex.

We see this everywhere: vagina size, penis size, ass size, how much we can take or not take, how much we want, and how our value is somehow intertwined with these objective facts and preferences. Isn't it exhausting enough to pay bills? Why do we add this extra layer on to sexuality?

There are certain social constructs and narratives we play over and over and over in our brains that are simply not true but have the power to deter us from being a fully realized, pleasure-focused hottie. And when we really think about it, they're morally bankrupt control tactics. These narratives are designed to make us feel bad about ourselves so we buy some product that is supposed to make us love ourselves.

Common Shame-Based Myths to Remove from Our Lives

BEWARE OF A LOOSE VAGINA.

The concept of having a loose vagina comes from society shaming women for having multiple sexual partners—but the biological concept of the vagina ever being loose is a complete myth. In their neutral state, the walls of any vagina are touching. The vagina is incredibly elastic (similar to the way the stomach can expand and contract after you eat), which allows it to stretch during sex and childbirth. While vaginas change over time, the idea that they become "loose" is a myth. Many companies have benefited from selling tightening creams and gels to make you feel "virginal" or tight for your partner's benefit, but all those do is constrict the skin, causing tears along the vaginal wall, making it super uncomfortable to do anything. Be nice to your vagina, if you have one, and remember that she/he/they is a self-cleaning babe whose elasticity should be celebrated.

VAGINAL DRYNESS IS BAD.

Vaginal dryness is inevitable on occasion, and it's nothing to be ashamed of. There are so many variables that can cause dryness, and it's not a reflection on your body or your ability or your partner's ability to turn you on. If you learn anything from this book, it needs to be that lubrication is your true best friend. A common concern of vulva owners is that they won't be able to take something or someone big inside of them. And yeah, I get that! But let me assure you that if you warm up, communicate, and use lube, you'll be fine. Warm up with fingers or a toy (with lube) so that the area (front hole = vulva, or back hole = anus) can get used to having something there! Add another finger, use a vibrator, get mentally aroused. Then try without fingers and lube. Your body needs prep before sticking something inside of it, and lubrication makes that process easier, sexier, and better!

PUBIC HAIR SHOULD BE REMOVED.

To shave or not to shave? That is the question! It is your decision to do with it as you like, as the idea that pubic hair is unclean is royally untrue. That tuft of hair is not only hot to play with and touch, but it's also there to reduce friction from outside elements (clothing, skin, other humans) and to protect your bits from any unnecessary bacteria. So the next time you're feeling around down there, touch how soft your pubic hair is. Really feel it. It's super sexy!

YOU CAN'T GET PLEASURE FROM ANAL PLAY.

Yes, you can masturbate anally! You, you, you, and you can all masturbate with your butt, no matter how you identify! It's such a hot way to get more connected to your body and to explore a new area that has a ton of nerve endings. In fact, anal masturbation is a great way to strengthen the sphincter muscles and create a deeper connection to genital health, and it feels so amazing to those out there with a prostate!

SOME NIPPLE SIZES ARE BETTER THAN OTHERS.

Dang, we've even shamed nipples. And for what? Because they all aren't small and pointing straight up? Nipples and the areola surrounding them are so sexy and perfectly normal at any size or shape, inverted or not!

YOU SHOULD HAVE PERFECT SKIN.

Some of us, many of us, have discolored skin that starts some-where on our inner thighs and leads right to the genitalia. It happens because our skin touches while we walk, because of the clothing we wear, and because of the sensitivity of our skin. Since this isn't seen or talked about in popular culture, this physical occurrence feels very insular and embarrassing. But, I promise you . . . you are not the only one! Maybe know-ing that will help us reclaim our power and not be fearful of letting it be seen!

FLACCIDITY ISN'T SEXY.

There is a lot of shame and stress placed upon penis owners of any identity, whether it's around size, cleanliness, owner-ship, or how hard or soft it is at any given time. But being hard doesn't mean you are aroused, and being soft doesn't mean you aren't! All bodies have the capacity to explore different aspects of sexuality without worrying about hardness or flac-cidness. You can please your partner and have sex, whether penetrative or not, with a soft or hard penis. Whatever you're bringing to the table is superhot.

ORGASMS AREN'T FOR YOU.

Anyone can have an orgasm! Orgasms aren't connected to partnered relationships, nor are they reliant on anyone besides yourself. A lot of our hesitancy about "being allowed" to experience touch, pleasure, sex, and orgasms is deeply rooted in how we have been taught to view sex and our bodies. No matter your relationship status, you should be having amazing orgasms on a regular basis. It's good for your mental and physical health—and for your sex life!

PHYSICALLY REMOVE SEXUAL SHAME WITH A RITUAL

Grab a piece of paper and write down all of the items you feel sexual shame over, such as the appearance of a specific body part; the sounds you make when having sex; a fetish, fantasy, or desire. Perhaps you feel shame over these things because society made you feel that way, or perhaps a former lover responded negatively to these things when you revealed this part of yourself to them. Be honest with yourself—no one else will see this. It might be difficult to even conjure the words—and that's OK, dear reader.

When you are done, take your piece of paper into the bathroom. Light a candle, shut off the lights, and look at yourself in the mirror.

Hold the paper and repeat: I will not feel shame because of the items on this list.

Repeat this 5 times or however many times feels good to you. Run the water from the sink. Light the paper with the candle, let the paper burn so it's touching some of the written words. (Not all the words! You don't want to burn yourself or start a house fire! Be safe in your ritual.) Place the paper under the running water and put out the flames. Grab some of the wet ashes and put them in the toilet. Pour the liquid candle wax into the toilet over the ashes. Say the phrase one more time . . . and flush. Sometimes the physical removal is all it takes to erase (or at least diminish) your feelings of shame. Repeat as needed.

MASTURBATION AS A GUIDE TO SELF-LOVE AND GREAT SEX

If you're reading this book, it's safe for me to assume that you're one of the following humans in the world:

1| A person with a deep need to update their body image.

2| A lovely human who wants to get more in touch with their own body and sexual pleasure.

3| A gorgeous being who is looking to understand their partner better and enhance their sex life.

4| A coffee-table book picker-upper. Good to see you here!

5| A hot lover who is deeply supportive!

No matter who you are or what your intentions for being here are, I'm happy you've made it this far. As we've moved through the book, I've asked you to be introspective, to reflect, and to use what you have learned to connect with your body and the pleasure you seek.

Now we're going to get physical. More physical than writing down pleasures, more physical than standing naked in front of the mirror and accepting our bodies (although I would argue that is incredibly physical when you take into account

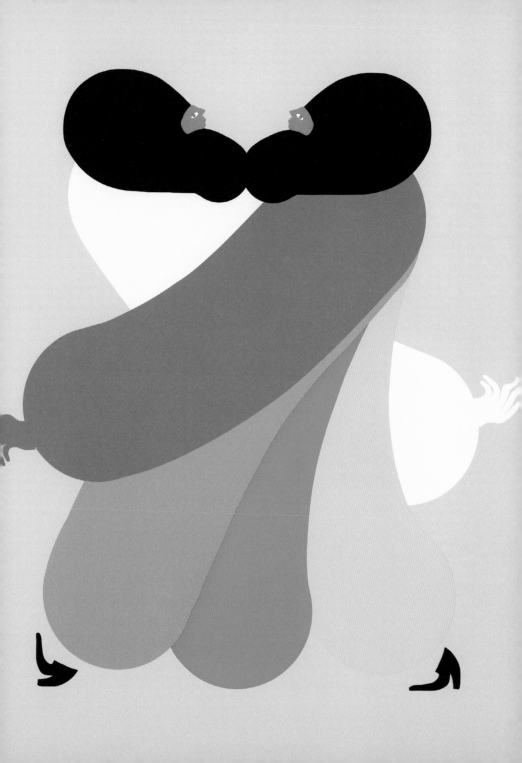

how connected our brains and bodies are). Today, I'm asking you to please yourself sexually (of course, if you consent).

Masturbation helps you feel more positive about your body. Not only does masturbation release a crazy amount of dopamine, endorphins, and oxytocin (love and bonding hormones), but it's also the best way to explore your body and get to know the types of touch that you do and don't enjoy. For example, have you ever touched your genitalia and it felt way too sensitive? Almost painful? Great—I mean, not great. Not great to feel pain when you don't want it. But now you know where you don't want to be touched. Note that masturbation can be more challenging for folks with body dysphoria—and whether or not that's true for you, maybe genital touching just isn't going to feel good for you. Consider this: The human body is covered in nerve endings, and pleasure can be derived from countless body parts depending on how they're touched. The chest, armpits, inner thighs, belly, and neck are all excellent places to explore on this journey.

Making decisions for yourself in the midst of solo play translates to you feeling more comfortable when you're making decisions about your body with a partner. If you can get yourself off, you can show a current or future partner how to get you off. You can also, for sure, tell your doctor you'd like a second opinion or ask your boss for a raise. Masturbation connects what you want internally to what you need externally.

It gives you the confidence to ask for what you want. It's an incredibly transferable skill set.

So, let's get to it. Buckle up, buttercup!

The Solo Play Practices

The next five activities are designed to get you moving, playing, and touching yourself in a way that makes you feel good. I, of course, can't tell what genitalia you have because I'm not a mind reader. So you move and stroke and rub and caress the way that works for you.

GET IN THE MOOD WITH A NONSEXUAL ACTIVITY

Make a playlist, light some candles, make an incredible dinner for yourself, take a hot shower, rub your feet, oil up your body, wear the hottest, most comfortable outfit you own.

The thing about masturbation is that it still holds a seat at the taboo table in popular culture. By creating a mood with day-to-day activities, it normalizes solo play so that you can begin without judgment and open up to the possibilities of exploring arousal and pleasure.

TASK: *Create a playlist filled with all the tunes you find calming or sexy, and play it when you're feeling particularly interested in masturbating. Maybe you've had a long workday. Use this play-list as you wind down and transition into a pleasurable moment with yourself.*

GIVE YOURSELF PERMISSION

It's right about the time when I'm oiling up my body where I'm like, "Laura, you're being ridiculous." But I know that this is my Inner Saboteur talking. Take a beat, drop into mindfulness, remember that you deserve it, and move forward with your solo playtime. Maybe it feels odd to have to give yourself permission to act on pleasure, but it's important. With all the messages you have internalized about your own body, all the oppression we have experienced and internalized, it's no wonder difficulties might arise when actually getting down to pleasure.

TASK: *While the music is playing and the candles are lit, find a quiet moment for yourself to feel your heart and listen to your breath. Your body is changing and reacting to your arousal, and that is the ultimate permission to allow yourself the pleasure you deserve.*

CREATE YOUR OWN TEMPLATE

I encourage you to create your own little nook in which to pleasure yourself—a pleasure station, if you will. Maybe this is your candlelit bathroom where you jerk, rub, or pat off in the shower, or maybe it's your bed where you surround yourself with tons of pillows. Whatever it is, find a place that makes you feel great.

TASK: *If you were to make little adjustments to your space that would make it easier to masturbate, what would you do? Would you keep the lubricant closer to the bed? Would you invest in a water-resistant throw blanket to use when masturbating? Make a list of those little upgrades and work your way toward creating your personal pleasure sanctuary.*

GO ALL EROTIC

Visual, audible, and readable stimulation are a natural part of solo play and can rev up the exploration you have with yourself. Plus, they allow you to play out any fantasies you're interested in while in the comfort of your own home.

TASK: *If interested—noting that not everyone will be into erotica, and that's OK—take a peek at a few sexy photos or listen to some erotic audio. Notice the physical changes your body experiences. Even better, watch your genitalia (perhaps in a mirror) when encountering an erotic stimulus—there is something really sexy about seeing your own body's arousal.*

THE BREATH AND PLEASURE CONNECTION

Breathwork is a technique where you intentionally change your breathing pattern to connect with your emotional, mental, and physical state. With masturbation, oxygen is a key player in promoting blood flow for arousal. But guess what: A lot of us stop breathing when we feel pleasure. We hold our breath, tighten up, and forget to check in with our core functions as humans. This can lower or even eliminate sensation to our most pleasurable parts.

TASK: *Focus on the breath when pleasuring yourself. Once you're getting into it and touching your genitalia, breathe into your stomach with every rub or stroke or pat. Instead of shallow or quick breaths, take in long breaths and exhale slowly. This will help regulate your heart rate, get enough oxygen to all the parts that need them, and boost arousal with every breath.*

The Body Is One Big Erogenous Zone

My goodness, reader, the body is super fascinating. The slightest touch in particular areas has the power to send shivers in all different directions. Genitalia often get all the credit, but there are other fleshy bits that can serve you well in solo play or in partnered sex. Meet the erogenous zones, parts of the body that excite sexual feeling when touched and stimulated.

Sensitive areas like the neck, forearms, inner thighs, and buttocks react to different types of touch and can build up your arousal to the point where you can't help but masturbate!

No matter where you are with masturbation—whether you're still working on conquering those mental blocks, or you're the ruler of your own masturbatorium—erogenous zones are great areas to explore in order to find or enhance your pleasure. But where to touch? That's up to you! Each area of the body will have a different sensation based on the type of touch it receives. Touch can be broken down into a few categories: rub, squeeze, caress, spank, pat, pinch, and lick.

RUB: *Nipples, Buttocks, Stomach, Inner Thighs, Back*

Oh yeah, give that butt a rub! Apply light pressure and try to match the motion with the in-and-out of your breath to connect more of your body to the experience—your genitals can't have all the fun!

SQUEEZE: *Breasts, Chest, Buttocks, Inner Thighs, Stomach*

Yep! Give your body a little squeeze! The sensation will draw blood to the area and make it more sensitive. This is a great opportunity to test your personal limits of how hard you like to be squeezed in those areas.

CARESS: *Neck, Nipples, Buttocks, Stomach, Inner Thighs, Back, Breasts, Chest*

Try lightly touching these areas with the tips of your fingers. Go slow and follow where your fingers take you!

SPANK: *Buttocks, Inner Thighs*

While you're vibing out and touching yourself, give your butt or thighs a little spank! Fun fact: Your pain tolerance is much higher when aroused, and that spank could be an excellent gateway to different types of erotic stimulation that isn't genitalia based. Plus, it's superhot!

PAT: *Nipples, Buttocks, Stomach, Inner Thighs, Back*

More than a rub, less than a spank, the pat can create an arousing sensation with a full-hand tap on the body, bringing blood to the surface and making the area much more sensitive.

PINCH: *Nipples*

With the pads of your fingers, give your nipples a little pinch. Press to your liking. Circular motions or pulling on the nipples can be arousing and deeply sensual.

LICK: *Everywhere*

With a flat or pointed tongue shape, you can create a unique sensation on different parts of your body. Of course, maybe you can't reach all the places—but if you can reach, go for it. A slight lick to the inner wrist can do wonders.

The Orgasm Section

Want to sleep better? Want to feel less anxious? Your wellness smoothie can't make you shake in pleasure, but an orgasm can.

An orgasm is, in the simplest terms possible, a release of erotic tension. From there, orgasms can vary wildly: For one, they can be felt in many different areas of the body, such as your toes or stomach. Sometimes they can be felt in waves. Sometimes they cause ejaculation. Sometimes an orgasm won't be the thing you're striving for!

Ah yes, you heard it here first. An orgasm is not the be-all and end-all solution to masturbation or sex, but it is a fantastic good time! When starting a masturbation journey with yourself, it's really easy to use orgasms as the marker for winning at pleasure. Taking time to really touch yourself, exploring what feels good, and considering all the different arousal points is way more productive than feverishly trying to reach an orgasm that may or may not be on the horizon. Pleasure is less about reaching a climax and more about enjoying the ride.

ORGASM PHASES

An orgasm can be broken down into four phases:

- EXCITEMENT: Feeling aroused? Feeling the pings in your genitalia? That's it!

- PLATEAU: Heavier breathing, clothes are off, you're touching, you're feeling—with or without another person.

- ORGASM: A burst of pleasure. Note: Everyone experiences orgasms differently. Maybe your orgasm feels like a release while others might experience a rolling orgasm experience.

- RESOLUTION: This is often categorized as feeling spent, like you're coming down from orgasm mountain— enjoy the ride.

Up the Ante

Want to go pro? There are many great ways to heighten your solo play night (or day) and take you over the pleasure edge and into the orgasm you're seeking. Here are some ideas to try:

EROTIC GELS OR STIMULANTS

These help promote blood flow to the genitals and increase stimulation. Try one out in your next solo sesh! They can be used by anyone, but do check the label to make sure the materials will not cause an allergic reaction for you! (More on this in chapter 4.)

WATCH YOURSELF MASTURBATE

I double dare you! But really, this is a great way to get to know your body more! Things change when you're aroused: Your skin may turn a different color, your genitalia might start to swell, your heart could start beating faster, your genitals might start to appear more wet. Take a mirror and really look at what you're doing down there—get your brain used to seeing how your body reacts when stimulated. Do you think Zac Efron ever has a masturbation session where he doesn't look at his genitals? No way.

GET ANAL!

Yes yes yes. As I said before, this is something you're allowed to try, feel good about, and get pleasure from! Whether you're by yourself or with a partner(s), it's important that you're in the right mindset and feeling sexy. Start by going slow and using lubricant. Use a finger or palm to circle around the pad of the anus and really get to know it. You will feel that the sphincter muscles expand and contract to your touch. You can wear a latex or nitrile glove to keep bacteria at bay. Or just wash your hands before and after.

The most common questions I get about anal sex are whether it's morally dirty or physically dirty ("poop comes from there!"). It's not—on both accounts. The morality of sex (of all kinds) is often deeply tied to the belief that sex is or should be solely for reproduction. Since anal sex doesn't have anything to do with human creation, it often gets a big, shameful wag of the finger—but this is pretty bogus. So please go forth and feel zero shame when exploring anal. As far as the physically dirty part, I would argue that there are things that are far less sanitary than having anal sex: We humans do things like touch subway poles and kiss our dogs on the nose (guilty on both counts). This isn't to say we shouldn't use necessary precautions like lube, condoms, and latex or nitrile gloves, but we can ease off from being scared of a little poop. Also note: If you're adult enough to play in that area, you should be adult enough to recognize its main function.

Self-pleasure is so cool and so important, and it is an emotionally transferable act: If you show yourself that you deserve pleasure, you're more willing to recognize the good you deserve in life. Keep going in your masturbatory journey and let it guide you, babes!

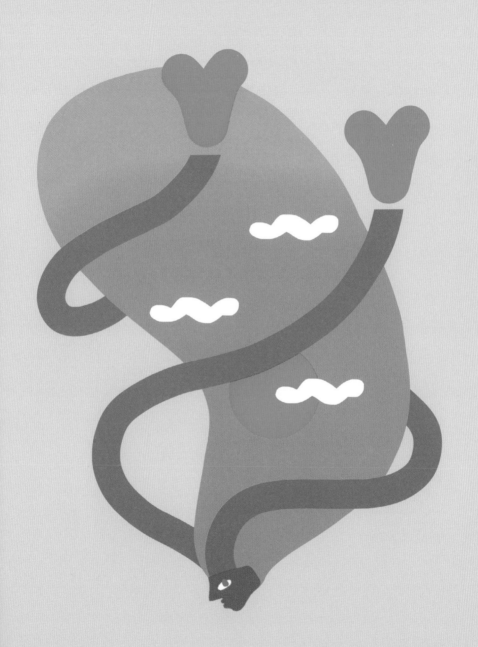

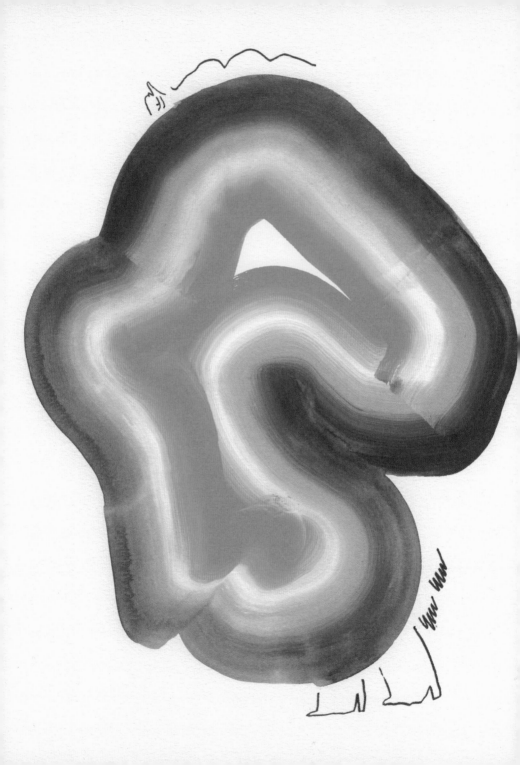

4

An Ode

to the

Sex Toy

Ah, yes. Sex toys.
The prized accessories
of getting off. I would
even go as far as saying
they have their own
magical powers.
Yep, you read it here
first: Sex toys are magic!

THE MAGICAL SEX TOY

First off, they have the literal power to change, revolutionize, and enhance both your solo and your partnered sex life. With every little or large buzz, thrust, plug, or spank, sex toys allow you to take control of your pleasure at any given time.

Secondly, sex toys give us a new range of motion to getting off. Sure, using our hands is cool, but not everyone has access to their genitalia via their appendages or even wants to use them to get off, considering that our skin is porous and we touch a lot of things throughout the day (*this may or may not be a PSA for washing your hands*). These buzzy, thrusty, ribby bits of design wonder make it easier to get off for some people and are an excellent tool for those who don't know what they like or how to communicate those needs.

Thirdly, and perhaps most important, sex toys are a physical manifestation of the autonomous pleasure you give to yourself. The personal power behind giving yourself an elevated form of pleasure has a direct and transferable connection to how you treat yourself on a day-to-day basis. Sex toys are to masturbation the way a steamy, saucy bowl of linguine is to a night of solo self-care. It just enhances the whole experience.

(Now I want linguine.)

Solo play aside, paying for and owning a sex toy is a big step in the journey of loving your body and having great sex. Even if you think it's silly or mundane or simply another day searching for dildos on the internet like you typically do (I see you, my dildo searchers), there is something very powerful about purchasing an object just for you.

Sex toys tend to bring out a bit of an "I do what I want" attitude among users—an incredibly transferable mindset that should be harnessed and adopted in everyday life. You did the research, you made the purchase, you gave the toy a home (maybe even a name), you use it when you want to get yourself off however you like: hence, "I do what I want." Now, imagine if every time you went out with friends, you decided when you wanted to head home for the night. Or every time you went to the doctor, you decided to ask for more context or seek a second opinion. Or even when you go to work—imagine you knew your worth at every turn and decided to ask for more compensation without ever hesitating. This is the magical power of masturbation and sex toys. You're giving yourself pleasure with a toy you picked out and purchased because you know you deserve it. When you intimately connect with yourself, that outlook can be applied to other areas of your life.

Good thing to note: A lot of sex toy packaging has wildly, unnecessarily gender-coded language. Some companies have expanded to include a more diverse range of human experiences, but often it's not the most representative of shopping experiences. I encourage you to look past the packaging to see if this toy and its functions will please you and your body.

As you work on recognizing how important it is to show yourself love, a vibrator, a cock ring, or even a paddle lying on your bed or in a dresser is a reminder that you are the omnipotent being that makes decisions for you.

All hail, _____!
(NAME HERE)

Sex Toy Q&A

WHAT IF I'M IN A RELATIONSHIP?

People inside and outside of a relationship still deserve a relationship with themselves and are allowed to use sex toys during solo or partnered sex! Sex toys don't equal cheating. Sex toys aren't a replacement for partnered experiences; they're an enhancement.

WHAT IF MY PARTNER DOESN'T WANT ME TO USE A SEX TOY?

I would prompt you to ask your partner why they feel this way and where that boundary comes from. They might be feeling replaced or inadequate by the very sight of a product that gives you pleasure. While it is not their right to impede your happiness at any turn, this is a great time to have better communication around sex and what you're both into. There are ways for you both to enjoy sex toys and even hotter moments where you both pick out sex toys for each other! Relationships are work and require communication in order to move forward. If your partner isn't being receptive to this kind of communication, then alas, my love, this is no partnership.

WHAT IF I GET USED TO IT?

There is a common misconception that using sex toys will ruin sex with a real human being. I find this to be wildly offensive and definitely a way to police human sexuality—and this kind of blatant sexism is often directed toward women. The underlying message here is that if you use a sex toy, your partner(s) will not be able to please you because you've gotten used to how good the vibrator/dildo/paddle/etc. is and they can't compete—which is totally, completely untrue.

WHAT IF I HAVE A PENIS OR A LARGE CLITORIS—CAN I STILL USE SEX TOYS?

Masturbation sleeves, cock rings, anal toys, dildos, and vibrators can all be used by people with external genitalia!

Vibration, pressure, and toy shapes and/or sizes are transferable and adaptable to anyone using it.

CAN I NUMB MY GENITALIA WITH VIBRATION?

I very much understand this concern around high vibration in a sensitive area. But there hasn't been any real evidence that links the two. If the vibration is too high, you may experience temporary numbness, making an orgasm difficult to reach. But in those cases, it's not long-term and you should turn the vibrator down for a bit so your genitalia can catch up to the sensation.

IS USING A SEX TOY FOR LONELY PEOPLE?

I can't even tell you the number of conversations I've had with people who felt that sex toys (and masturbation, in general) were only for lonely people. Let me be very, very, very clear: Owning a sex toy is so positive and perfect. It's for the single, the dating, the partnered, the coupled, the messing around, and the not searching for anyone (ANYONE!). In other words, it's for everyone and anyone who needs it. It's beautiful and glorious. You have to find your own path, of course, but hopefully by the end of this chapter, you will be well on your way.

IF I, A CISGENDER STRAIGHT MAN, USE AN ANAL TOY, WILL THAT MAKE ME GAY?

No, it won't. Anal pleasure will not make you gay. Sexual orientation is about who you are attracted to, not what you do (or fantasize about doing) with them sexually. People like who they like and are free to do what they like with each other. If you want to have anal pleasure with yourself or another person, amazing! You should try it! It doesn't affect how you identify.

The Rules Around Sex Toy Ownership

1| Sex toys do not take the place of partners because sex toys can't provide emotional or physical connection. No sex toy has ever acted out a sexual fantasy of mine and then brought me ice cream afterward. Facts.

2| Sex toys are for everyone—not just for single people. Sex toys can be used by yourself or with your partner(s), no matter your relationship status.

3| Sex toys can't change your sexual orientation.

4| Sex toys are not immoral, pathetic, sad, or any other synonymous word for negative.

5| No matter who you are, sex toys are there to make sexual stimulation more fun, more accessible, and more exciting. (Although the sex toy industry has a long way to go before people with a disability are fully included in the marketing and design of their products. See Access Is Key on page 136.)

FACT: Sex toys can be used by anyone of any sexual orientation, gender, body type, body shape, body size, or genitalia. They are universal tools designed for pleasure—the foremost inclusive products on the market. Of course, marketing around these toys would have us believe that vibrators are solely for vulva owners and cock rings are only for penises, but really, sex toys are there for you to play with and enjoy. Personal creativity should not be limited by misguided marketing.

Access Is Key

Our accessibility and comfort should be taken into consideration when choosing a quality product designed for pleasure. Not everyone will be able to perfectly grip around a toy, lay on their back, rest on their front, reach, bend, squat, stretch, sit on, or stand up in order to get off. We all have various ways we experience accessibility, and our sex toys should work for us—not against us.

People with mobility challenges or physical differences are often removed from the pleasure conversation, and that's a pretty big shame. While mainstream sex toy marketing hinges on these products being an added bonus to a "normal" sex life (already problematic), sex toys and sex technology are an empowering way to make sex accessible. Products like thigh strap-ons, flexible massagers, toy mounts, sex tools, Kegel products, slings, and stackable rings to modulate penetration depth are all designed to make sex more accessible to more people.

But while sex technology is a useful tool, it's important to note the connection between disability and poverty. Expendable income to purchase a sex toy with all the bits and bobs can be out of the question. Financial privilege is very, very real—and the sex toy industry can sometimes feel like only people with that privilege can access high-quality toys. I want to reassure you, reader, that a satisfying sex toy doesn't have to break the bank. A good sex shop has a dedicated, trained staff who can help pick out a toy in your budget that is made of high-quality materials, doesn't have any toxins (like some lower-cost toys do), and can give you the pleasure you're looking for. Economical sex toys with hands-free or self-activating motions (meaning, you don't have to be holding it for it to work) are also available and worth the research. You deserve the insight on how to choose the toy best suited for you and your needs, at whatever price.

MATERIALS, CHEMICALS, AND WHY IT'S IMPORTANT TO READ THE LABEL

The material of a sex toy is incredibly important to how your genitalia experiences pleasure and also how you make good decisions for your pleasure-seeking body. There is little regulation on the materials that can be used in sex toys, and unfortunately, companies have used this as an opportunity to sell cheap toys to consumers who don't know any better. So when a customer complains about irritation when using the product, the company doesn't have to live up to the consequences of that complaint because genital irritation can be caused by many different factors.

The major reason there is little regulation is because we still see sex toys and their use as shameful and, therefore, we don't give the industry the proper attention it deserves. There are a lot of sex toy companies out there that are doing it right, but there are some that are still raking in money off the lack of education provided about sex toys. It is on us to figure out which toys are best for our bodies.

- Cost-efficient doesn't equal toxic, and expensive doesn't equal nontoxic. Toys come in many different price ranges across the toxic and nontoxic spectrum. Do some research and read the ingredients on the label before purchasing a sex toy.

- Phthalates are a common chemical found in sex toys to make them softer and more flexible. Long-term phthalate exposure has been linked to cancer and is incredibly harmful to all reproductive systems. Because phthalates are active materials, they leak out of the toy and into the body, disrupting hormone balance and reproductive functions.

- If a toy smells like chemicals, or has a fruit smell, put a condom on it while using it or get rid of it. Most of these toys are made of PVC plastic or jelly materials, which are toxic. The fruit smell is usually there to cover up the chemical smell—fun. Because our skin is porous and genitalia contain mucous membranes, the chemicals in toys can enter the body and cause damage. Note: While it's easy to say "just get rid of those sex toys," it's not economically sound to constantly be buying new toys in case the one you have doesn't meet safety standards. Using a condom over sex toys can alleviate that concern. Or, consider saving up for a higher-quality toy or shopping around for a less expensive, safer toy!

- Science experiment: If you put two sex toys with active materials (i.e., materials with toxic ingredients and additives) next to each other, they will bind together over time . . . an odd sight to find at the bottom of your sex toy drawer.

Sex Toy Materials

THE GOODS

These materials are nonactive, nonporous (don't hold bacteria), and made of the same material your family swears by for cookware—and now you'll never forget that piece of info!

- Medical-grade, pure silicone

- Glass/Pyrex

- Stainless steel

THE OKAYS

These materials are safe to use with the caveat that people with more sensitive skin might find them irritating, as they require solvent-free, phthalate-free varnishes.

- Wood

- ABS plastic

- Crystal/natural stone

- Elastomer

THE NOT-OKAYS

These materials are known to be active, carcinogenic, and impossible to clean, as they hold bacteria (porous). The recommendation here is to reconsider the toy altogether or place a condom over it when in use.

- TPE

- TPR

- Cyberskin

- Jelly rubber

- PVC and vinyl

- Hard plastic

TYPES OF SEX TOYS

There are so many different types of sex toys out there, including internal and external toys, ones that have nothing to do with genitalia, and ones that take pleasure to a whole new level. Before we start, I must tell you: There is no such thing as the best sex toy. Whenever anyone learns about my body image/sexual wellness life, they always ask me, "What is the best sex toy out there?" Honestly, I can't answer that. There are expensive toys. There are economical toys. There are toys that thrust and bend, there are toys that stay in position, and there are toys you have to manually operate. It all depends on what you like.

- ANAL BEADS provide a unique sensation when each bead is inserted into the anus. Some people really enjoy slowly removing each bead during orgasm so that the sphincter muscle ripples on contact.

- ANTERIOR FORNIX EROGENOUS ZONE (A.K.A. A-SPOT) TOYS are longer versions of clitoral urethral vaginal complex toys (see following) and are designed to pleasure the patch of tissue at the top of the vaginal tube between the cervix and the bladder—it's all the way back there!

- BULLETS/POCKET ROCKETS are small, finger-size, vibrating toys designed for external use and great for anyone who likes more direct stimulation.

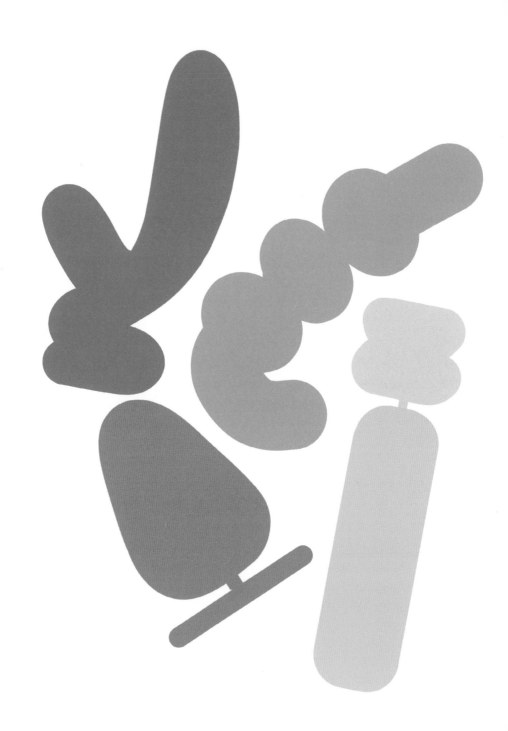

- CLITORAL URETHRAL VAGINAL COMPLEX (A.K.A. G-SPOT) TOYS are curved, hard toys that put pressure on the spongey wall inside the vagina that sends pleasure along the clitoral complex. (Note: *Clitoral urethral vaginal complex* is a relatively new term that represents a sort of wall that connects the vagina, the urethra, and parts of the clitoris—once known as the G-spot.)

- COCK RINGS are circular items made of silicone, jelly, elastomer, and sometimes steel that go around the base of outer genitalia or dildos. It's designed to keep blood inside the penis without having it escape back out, and to keep dildos in place in a harness. Some cock rings even have vibrators attached to them for extra fun! Cock rings without give (i.e., steel and hard silicone) do need a circumference size in order to play safe and not cause priapism—unwanted, persistent erection lasting more than 4 hours (it's very painful). If you're unsure, consider ones with an elastic or snap-release band!

- DILDOS are phallic-shaped objects used for sexual stimulation. Some are shaped like penises, some look like nondescript wands, and some even look like fantasy cocks (I'm talkin' ones shaped like hookah bellows). These can be used internally in front holes and back holes, but make sure to use one with a flared base for back hole/anal play.

- GLASS AND METAL WANDS are nonporous, sleek, non-vibrating pieces that could possibly be confused for art. These can be used on vagina owners or for anal play. They're great for anyone looking for deep internal pleasure; slower, more steady dilation; or temperature play. Plus, glass is known to be an incredibly affordable and body-safe material when searching for sex toys on a budget.

- MASTURBATION SLEEVES (A.K.A. STROKER TOYS) are designed to simulate oral, anal, or vaginal sex inside their encapsulated cylinder.

- PLUGS are anal toys with a large surface connected to a thinner stem and then a flared base. They are perfect for people looking to start anal play and experiment with size. They are used for anal pleasure.

- P-SPOT (PROSTATE) TOYS are curved toys designed to put pressure on the prostate. These toys were actually not invented for pleasure! They were created to push prostatic fluid through the urethra and out of the body for medical reasons. But, if you have a prostate, it also feels really good to do!

- RABBIT TOYS (A.K.A. TWO-IN-ONE TOYS) have an internal component and an external, usually vibrating, piece that provides double the pleasure.

- SEX CHAIRS and ramps support sex play and make it easier to access different parts of the body without strain. These tools can be for anyone but especially benefit people who experience mobility issues or need more support to hold parts of their body. As a plus-size woman, I find that ramps make it a lot easier for me to position myself comfortably and gain access to my genitalia without feeling frustrated by having a belly or larger thighs. These tools are here for you to experience pleasure in the most body-friendly way—it's totally OK and perfectly wonderful to use accommodations to improve your pleasure.

- SEX SWINGS are suspended harnesses that allow partners to move freely during intercourse—and if you can find a New York apartment that allows for this setup to be mounted into the beams, you let me know.

- SLIMLINE TOYS are typically hard plastic, shaped like an elongated cone, and a simple (but very good) product. These toys are for front-hole internal use and external use only. (All toys used for anal play need to have a flared based so that they don't get pulled into the rectum by the anus's sphincter muscles.) Depending on the material, these can be great couples' toys!

- WAND OR MASSAGER TOYS have a larger surface area and a handle (stem) that allows for multiple motors, and are perfect for all-over stimulation. They are designed for external use only.

A lot, right? And this is just a preliminary list! There are dual-stimulation sex toys, toys that will suck on your nipples, and toys designed to spank you! The fun part is researching, exploring, and understanding what you like so that you are more connected to your pleasure and, in turn, have quality communication with the lovers in your life. Sex toys provide a fantastic sense of autonomy. It's on you to figure out what you're into—through a laborious trial-and-error process, oh gosh!

Direct vs. Indirect Pleasure

Some people like very direct stimulation while others like it to be more indirect—this can vary on different parts of your body. For example, I'm very, very sensitive during external genital stimulation but I have a high, high pain tolerance on my body. The only way I know this is by trying things out, testing the intensity, and understanding my boundaries. Take some time and try putting vibration (or your fingers) on different parts of your genitalia. Try going directly on your clit, head of penis, or anus (insert the term you use for your body). Does that feel like too much? Try a different location. Do the same thing with skin sensation. Give yourself a good spank. On a scale of 1 to 10, with 10 being terribly painful and 1 being not at all, where would you place that? Find your thresholds and explore them, babes, but remember—your pain tolerance increases when aroused. Your pain rating may shift depending on your mood, and that's perfectly normal.

Two Toys at the Same Time

We're often lured in by the idea that one sex toy is able to do everything for us with the flip of a battery-operated switch. There are biological pieces to the solo play puzzle—different body parts require different stimulation, which can't all be achieved by one single toy. Internal nerve endings (front hole and anus) are more spread out and respond better to pressure rather than vibration. External nerve endings (clit, frenulum, whatever you like to call your external parts) are compact and get pleasure from rhythm, vibrations, tapping, licking, and sucking. Which means you might need or want to try using two toys at the same time.

HOW TO FIND THE TOY FOR YOU

Finding the perfect sex toy for you is kind of like finding the perfect running shoe. It needs to be comfortable and durable. It has to work with your body and any of its lovely quirks. While it doesn't need to be your favorite color, it is fun to match your new running shoe to your personality. Sex toys are the same except they're going on your genitals and not your feet (though that can also be pretty fun if you're adventurous).

The first sex toy I ever owned was a Barbie-pink, one-battery pocket rocket that only required a twist for it to start up. When I first looked at it, I laughed and swore to my friend who gave it to me that I would never use it. I think I might have even said, "This is never going near my vagina!" But when I went home, I stared at the toy, knowing it would elevate masturbation if I just gave it a try. So I did. I added the AA battery, turned the mechanism to the right, and placed it on my clit. Sure, it felt good after I maneuvered it around my belly and found the perfect spot on my genitalia where the vibration didn't feel too intense to experience. I can't speak for everyone, but I'm sure this might be one of those ubiquitous masturbation experiences that many a vulva owner has had: It was fun, but also it was just . . . fine.

We're not going for fine, people. You have one life and you deserve to have the best orgasms imaginable in that life. Now, there are plenty of people who own pocket rockets and love them for a host of different reasons. But there are some, like myself, who find them cumbersome and difficult to use. Sex toys are a personal kind of purchase.

It takes some time and research to figure out which sex toy works for you. The most popular, most expensive, most technologically advanced toys out there might not gel with how your body operates. Everyone's body and sexual responses are different. But trust me, it's worth finding it! Finding a good sex toy will take your pleasure to the next level. It's also a significant milestone in your journey to self-love. As we've learned, loving yourself doesn't just come from looking in a mirror and exclaiming that everything is going to be great. It comes from making good decisions for yourself and your body, and choosing a toy that works for you physically and mentally is an important step. Instead of asking, "Which is the best sex toy?" ask, "Which is the best sex toy for me?"

> **Dear Reader**, I am a big fan of wand vibrators because the length of the handle makes it easier to hold during sex and even better during masturbation because I can navigate it around my body without putting too much strain on my shoulders and arms when reaching for my genitalia—a common occurrence with the aforementioned pocket rocket. But that's just me—I'm a wand queen, always have been and always will be.

WHAT TO ASK YOURSELF BEFORE PURCHASING A SEX TOY Of course, sex toy purchases can take some trial and error in order to find the perfect toy(s) for you. Consider these questions as you embark on your search!

- Are there any materials to be cautious of? Do you have any allergies?

- What is your budget? Sex toys come in a wide range of price points—the most expensive doesn't always mean the best!

- Battery operated? Rechargeable? Is the power source important to your purchase?

- What kind of pleasure do you like? Internal? External? Front? Back? Vibration? Pressure?

- If vibration is your game, do you want something with a wider surface area on your genitalia or something more direct and pinpointed with a smaller surface area?

- Should you consider accessibility in this purchase? Would it be better to purchase a toy that doesn't require strain in any extremity?

- Does this toy need to be waterproof, splashproof, or submergible for any hot tub play or squirters?

Still not sure? That's totally fine! There are plenty of reasonably priced toys that have multiple functions for users to try.

TAKE PLEASURE FURTHER

In the previous chapter, we learned the importance of masturbation as a tool to feel more connected with our self and our needs. We talked about how to remove the shame we often associate with the act and with our body. Let's take that a little further by considering, in the most indulgent way possible, what you would need right now to have the most incredible orgasm. How can you incorporate your sex toy? How can you push it even further?

HAVE A MASTURBATION DATE WITH YOURSELF AND YOUR SEX TOY: We covered this in the last chapter, but now we're looking to elevate it a little more. Mix things up! Try masturbating in a different position where you can experience hands-free pleasure. Maybe nipples are involved? What if you tried a plug with the OG solo play moves you have down? Try it out and see how it feels. Maybe write about the experience.

CREATE A HOT FANTASY: Throughout your day, really build up a fantasy for yourself. Where are you? Who is there? What is happening? Try not to shame yourself for what is going on in your head . . . you might find that your brain will lead you to something you never thought about. Now that you've been teasing yourself with the fantasy, create it for yourself with your sex toy(s) and/or partner(s)!

PLAY WITH THE OTHER PARTS: Give yourself a little smack on the ass, pinch a nipple, grab your sides, or brush yourself up against a cold surface (hello, refrigerator). Play with the other erogenous zones to see whether that takes sex toy time a little further.

DESIGN A MOOD: Light and color have an incredible effect on your mood, the same way that putting on a fresh outfit—or hot Rihanna lingerie—can give you a confidence boost. What are the sexiest mood-setting modifications you can do for yourself?

WRITE IT ALL DOWN: Who says you can't create a little erotica for yourself? In your notebook, write your own erotic story. Next time you're looking to get in the mood, you can read it, or continue writing the story in installments over time!

Oh, hey! How are you doing? I know, I know. I'm asking you to write things down and go sex toy shopping—more homework from the author. We have already spoken about loving your body, finding pleasure, and having great solo sex, but the hot sex or orgasms aren't a stopgap just because you have found one thing that works. More things work! Right now, we're connecting that body love we learned about with tangible action. Feeling like it's too much? Take a second, and continue when you're ready.

PARTNERS AND SEX TOYS

There is honestly nothing better than getting in bed with a person who is jazzed to use all the tools necessary to bring you to an earth-shattering orgasm. Praise be to those humans! Using sex toys with a partner is superhot and can really heighten the overall experience as you both explore different types of stimulation together. However, pulling out a sex toy without having a conversation first is also not helpful.

If you'd like to introduce sex toys into your partnered sex life, you need to have a conversation with your partner. Here are some pointers:

- THERE ISN'T A PERFECT MOMENT—just have the conversation. There isn't a perfect moment in a relationship or situationship to bring up the topic of sex toys or to introduce your sex toy chest in the bedroom. I get it: We're afraid of scaring off our partners. This is where

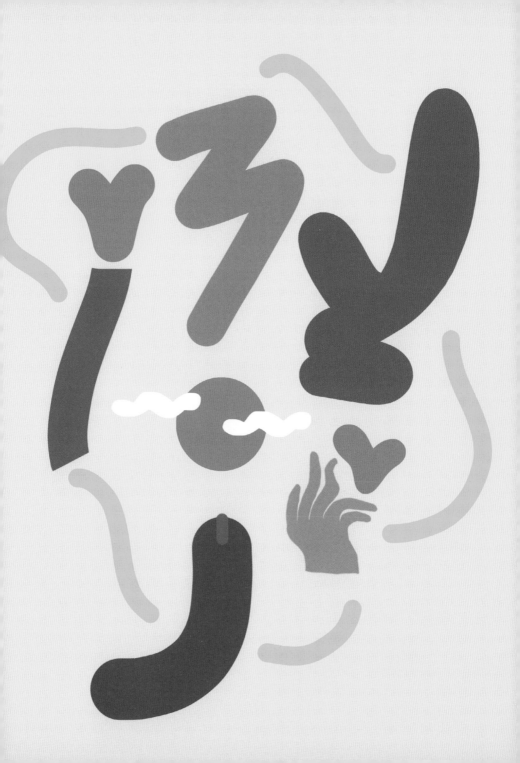

communication is the forever and always best tool—
have a conversation before you get into the bedroom.

- KEEP THE NEUTRALITY. Everything that you're doing and/
or proposing is perfectly normal. Using sex toys in bed
with a partner or on a partner is super fun. Approach
it as if you're talking about what to eat or what Netflix show you're going to watch or some other neutral
conversation topic . . . just be chill.

- REASSURANCE IS SOMETIMES NEEDED. Look, we as a society
need to be more comfortable with how we experience
pleasure in a safe and healthy way, but until we get
there, we must remember that we've all been taught
to hate our bodies and to feel shame around sex. It
might come up that your partner feels insecure that
they can't please you in the same way as a sex toy.
This is a totally understandable feeling. Hold space
for your partner, reassure them, and be kind in your
exploration.

- NOT ALL TOYS NEED TO BUZZ. Maybe playtime with your
partner means an erotic massage oil, a paddle, or a
butt plug. Sex and sex toys are all about you and what
you like. They are what comes after a boundary-
setting conversation. They are a means to an orgasm
your way. Your body, always your choice.

- TRANSFERRABLE SEX TOYS. Most sex toys can be used across genitalia and bodies—of course, first consider the material and your comfort level around sharing—which makes them an excellent tool to have when playing with your lover (again this word). I challenge you to think outside the box with sex toys and how they can be incorporated; consider putting a vibrator on your cheek during oral sex or experience a double penetration fantasy if you are a vulva owner when playing with a person who has a penis and a dildo. There are also remote-operated toys: One person wears it while the other one controls it (get consent, of course). Finding sex toys that both parties can use and play with changes the dynamic and makes everything a bit more fun.

Lubrication 101

Lube lube lubity lube.

I love lubrication. I love everything about it. There has not been a day in my sexual history where I've run out of lube, because I stockpile it as if the supply chain will cease to exist one day. Some people hoard paper towels; I will live off my throne of high-quality, water-based lubricants.

This was not always the case. I used to feel really self-conscious about using lubrication (maybe some of you can relate). How many times did I not ask for it, secretly apply it while my sex partner wasn't looking, or hide it in my wallet just in case I needed some on a date? And for what? Because I was scared of being judged.

Sadly, we have been widely taught that the need for lubrication somehow equates to your age, your vitality, or your body not working correctly—but in reality, needing lubrication just means you need lubrication. That's it. During sexual arousal, the vulva and clitoris swell while the vagina produces a clear-ish, wet substance biologically designed to reduce any kind of friction.

However, this response to sexual excitement can differ from person to person. Sometimes this wetness has nothing to do with arousal and everything to do with hormone levels or the glands in the cervix producing fluid to keep the vagina clean. Sometimes, stress or medication or hydration will affect the amount of wetness that happens. And sometimes, you can be really aroused and not wet at all. Dryness is a real thing that happens to every single person with a front hole/vulva. It doesn't matter your age or how fertile you are or any other reason that makes vulva-owning people feel bad about their bodies. It's really an individual experience.

Dear Reader, I used to believe every single negative thing about the use of lubrication, and that made me feel really bad about my body. Once, a sexual partner looked at me after I applied lube to a sex toy we were using and said, "Are you not into me?" It made me think something was wrong with me, that I wasn't working properly. I would always feel bad that my body wasn't good enough to produce the "regular" amount of wetness needed. As I've gotten older and more into sex education, I've come to learn that natural wetness isn't the be-all and end-all of personal arousal.

If you only take away one thing from this book, let it be this: Lubrication is a necessary part of using sex toys and having sex. Lubrication is really your best friend in all forms of pleasure. It makes genitals more sensitive, slicker, and easier to please. Nobody wants dry skin against dry skin. Whether it's foreplay, oral sex, penetrative sex, solo sex, or anything else, lubrication plays a hot role.

Spit is not lube. Excuse the blunt delivery, but I cannot explain to you how many times I've had to say this to friends, customers, exes, lovers. Spit doesn't attach itself to the mucous membranes along the vaginal wall, and therefore doesn't provide any lubrication during any form of penetration. In fact, spit dries out faster than lube and creates friction. This friction causes irritation in the form of nicks and tears in that area, making you more susceptible to harmful microbes entering the body—not fun. In sum, spit is not a replacement for lube.

But let me be clear: Spit can be very hot. Like, oh so hot. Like, spit in my mouth hot—if that's something you're into! The idea of using spit as a form of power play with consenting adults is really sexy. This is where you make decisions for your body and pleasure. Weigh the pros and cons of spit on your genitalia.

If spit is your thing, amazing. (Just don't use it instead of lube.) If spit is not your thing, there are simple ways to have that conversation.

PERFECTLY FINE RESPONSES IF YOUR PARTNER SUGGESTS USING SPIT AS LUBE

- "Spit isn't lube."

- "Spit is a slightly more viscous saliva, and saliva is quickly absorbed!"

- "I didn't consent to spit."

- "Spit on my face. I only use high-quality lubrication on my genitalia."

- "I don't put spit on my skin when it's feeling dry. Why would I put it on my genitalia?"

- "AHHH! While I really like spit play, I would love to use lubrication to reduce penetrative friction."

- "Would you use spit on Zac Efron?"

Some Lubes Are Better
Than Others

Just like sex toys, lubrication ingredients are very important to how we experience pleasure and feel comfort. And unfortunately, like sex toys, there are some ingredients that cause more harm than good. This is the lube that leaves you feeling sticky and tacky, that will bring about a certifiable yeast infection, or that, for some reason, tastes like cherries but insists on the label it can be used in any orifice. Babe, it just can't be.

INGREDIENTS TO AVOID

- ANYTHING FLAVORED: Flavored lubes have sweeteners, and just like glycerin, they are a quick ticket to Yeast Infection Land.

- BENZOCAINE: This is a numbing agent that removes sensation from the area to prolong a sexual experience or to decrease the pain associated with anal sex. Pain is there for a reason—to signal that something is wrong. There are better, safer, healthier ways to work through hypersensitivity and anal sex.

- GLYCERIN: Basically, it's a sweetener. And sweeteners don't belong in wet, porous places because they get sticky and tacky and can cause infections!

- MICROBICIDE NONOXYNOL-9: This ingredient is a spermicide, which seems dope but in fact can cause infections and increases your risk of STIs because of how easily it can travel through the body. Most companies do not use this ingredient because the risks far outweigh the benefits, but it's good to know what to look for!

- PARABENS AND PRESERVATIVES: Parabens and preservatives are used by food, cosmetic, and pharmaceutical companies to make products last for long stretches of time. Both have been connected to breast cancer and early puberty, as they mimic estrogen and hormone levels in the body.

- PETROLATUM: It suffocates your pores, making it difficult for your vulva to self-clean.

BUT, LAURA . . . WHY WOULD COMPANIES USE THESE INGREDIENTS?

Well, that's a good question. You would think that humans are generally kind and dedicated to making products with quality ingredients that allow everyone to partake in a cycle of doing good. But alas, that is far from true. There are a lot of companies that profit off the irritation, illness, and overall pain of the consumer. For example, getting a yeast infection might mean you purchase another product from the same overlord company to alleviate that irritation. Whether it's plain ignorance, being able to skirt around regulations because lawmakers turn a blind eye to sex-related products, or a desire to make more money off the results of bad ingredients, companies don't always use healthy, safe ingredients. Which is why it's important for us to research and understand what is being put on and inside our bodies. Also make sure to check the labels and expiration dates on items like lube and condoms so they are not being used past the recommended date.

Types of Lubrication

WATER-BASED

Water-based lubricant is great for front-hole and anal play, it washes off easily, and it won't stain your sheets! However, because it's water-based, it will need to be reapplied often, as it will dry up—but that's actually a really good trait, as it won't stay on top of the skin and hold bacteria. Water-based lubricant is safe to use with latex and non-latex gloves, dental dams, and condoms; it is digestible in the case of oral sex; and it is safe to use with all toy materials.

SILICONE-BASED

Silicone-based lubricant can be used for both front-hole and anal play. It's especially good for anal use because it lasts a long time. I would caution against front-hole use if the user has sensitive skin. Even though silicone-based lubricant is hypoallergenic and doesn't evaporate, it can collect bacteria if not properly washed away. Silicone-based lubricant can be used on most sex toy materials EXCEPT silicone toys. Silicone and silicone bind together over time and create a used-eraser texture on your sex toy. It is digestible but not very tasty—and it will stain your sheets and/or wooden dressers.

OIL-BASED

Oil-based lubricant is good for anal sex. Stay clear of front-hole sex because it's difficult to clean and can lead to bacterial vaginosis. It can double as a massage oil but will absolutely stain your sheets if you're not careful (invest in a waterproof sheet). A MUST-KNOW: Oil-based lubricants can only be used with non-latex condoms. Oil-based lube will break latex condoms.

HYBRID-BASED

Hybrid-based lubricants are a combination of both water-based and silicone-based lubricant, giving it a milky silk look. It's great for anal and front-hole play and contains a low amount of silicone, so it's safe to use with silicone toys. Hybrid-based lubricants are digestible and safe to use with all condoms.

NATURAL LUBRICANTS

I love unrefined coconut oil as an alternative to consumer packaged lubricants; however, I'd make this an alternative rather than a starting player. While products like coconut oil and olive oil hold a lot of the same benefits as regular lubricants, they can disrupt the vulva's pH balance, causing yeast infections. Also, as noted earlier, oil-based products are directly linked to breaking down latex.

CHOOSE THE RIGHT LUBRICANT FOR YOU Let's go on a lubrication adventure, shall we? Let's consider which lubricants we should and should not be using on our bodies. Be proud of your lube use! Maybe you'll even start carrying around a lube packet in your wallet or bag.

- First, be active in your sexual wellness. Read ingredients in the lubricants you're considering and weigh your options.

- Take into consideration your genitalia. What are they like? Are they sensitive? Do they feel drier on certain days? I know I ask a lot of questions throughout this book, but the reason is because I want you to connect with yourself! And in this case, your genitalia must be front and center in your decision-making.

- Will you be using a condom with this lubricant? If so, consider non-oil-based lube so that the latex doesn't deteriorate. Maybe throw a condom in that wallet or bag, as well!

- If you're able to, head to a local sex shop and feel the sample lubricants on your hand. Each has a different viscosity, slipperiness, smell . . . and even taste. Yep, tasteless lube is great for oral sex if your mouth tends to get dry! Of course, there are the flavored lubes that taste great, but definitely have a conversation with your partner about them to make sure they won't cause an infection.

- Practice not apologizing for needing lube. I would even go as far as saying you should try this in the mirror. Get used to saying, "Let me grab the lube," or "Can you put some lube on?" or even "Lube me up, baby!" Take up space in this world, and let that confidence run through everything you touch.

Let's Talk Pornography

Ooohhhh

Ahhhhhh

Poorrrnnnnoooo

The early foray into so much of our sexual enlightenment often includes the hush-hush yet wildly enticing genre known as pornography. Maybe it was the Playboy Channel. Maybe it was Skin-a-Max (Cinemax). Maybe it was a *Hustler* found in a parent's dresser. Maybe it was the internet! No matter what it was, porn has a rightful place in our sexual history as a first-time arousal point. I believe that pornography, erotica, nudie mags, audio porn, and all types of erotic-ness deserve to be on the leaderboard of sexual stimulus.

I love porn. Here I am admitting it to you, dear reader. I love the mainstream, the amateur. I love thinking about how long it took the creators to shoot one pool scene. Honestly, how did they shoot in the water? But more than loving porn itself, I love understanding the dynamics of pornography and how they affect us. Everything about porn has always been wildly fascinating to me. The more I've learned, the more interesting the world of porn has become. Porn is a great way to understand culture, trends, beauty standards, the connection between what people actually want and how they get it, and, sadly, who gets treated better according to the American value system.

A lot of us grow up hating our bodies, never looking in the mirror, finding it difficult to feel sexy within our own skin. And the closest thing we have to a tangible, sexual experience in that inadequacy is porn. It's so easy to access.

Just as exposure therapy is to loving your body, porn is to self-pleasure. The full gambit of erotic arts, in fact, is sexual terrain for discovering more ways to give yourself pleasure. And porn can be an excellent way to become more comfortable with your fantasies, inspire you to try new things, or even discover new sexual interests.

Though porn has its issues, which we'll discuss shortly, don't swear it off! It's a useful tool on your journey to self-pleasure and great sex. We simply need to remember that porn presents a fantasy, in the same way that every TV show you watch is a fantasy—yes, my dear reader, even the reality shows are a fantasy. These shows, like porn, are designed to incite emotion. But babe, we're in real life, where we pay bills, go to the doctor, date around, and have to pick out outfits for our cousin's wedding. And in real life, we deserve consent and respect. If you're finding that you or a sexual partner is nonconsensually adding aggressive porn performances to sexy time, take a step back from this learned behavior and reconnect to what you and the other person actually want and why.

LAURA'S PORNO HISTORY

I remember being in my teens and first discovering *Real Sex* on HBO. It was enthralling—so many types of people doing so many different things that I had never even thought possible. There was an entire episode about people into pony play! It was so cool! When I told a friend about it, she mentioned that she found a magazine called *Playboy* in her parents' garage; we immediately went and looked at it. Not long after, I came across one of those late-night faux porn films where the actors alluded to sexual activity but never actually used their genitalia. The scene began with a woman wearing a red dress next to her broken-down car in the middle of the Nevada desert. A man on a motorcycle rode past only to suddenly turn around and help her. But he did more than just help her! To remember it is to remember the '90s—the hair, the clothes, the convertible, the references to *Showgirls*.

Should I have seen those scenes at that age? No.

Do I regret it? No.

At the time, I had no idea what was happening with my body, and I had no idea that it was OK to touch myself. I was fortunate to come across sexual content that was consensual and positive. It was quite a remarkable discovery to a kid without any context.

Let's Discuss the Bad Parts of Porn

It is important for me to speak about pornography in this book with the utmost respect as well as a critical eye. I would be remiss if I just wrote, "PORN IS GREAT!" and left it at that. The truth is, not all porn is great. Not all porn is made fairly. Not all porn is ethical. Not all porn is anti-racist. Not all porn is about the celebration of human sexuality and sensuality. As someone who has spent a good deal of time working in the media industry, I believe that any form of entertainment and communication deserves a look-see with the highest form of critique. Before you click around on your favorite porn site, it's extremely important to remember that there are larger issues at play. Be considerate of what you consume and how that fits into your sexual journey!

- Porn categories are demoralizing and reduce humans to type, such as BBW, Asian, MILF, Ebony.

- Porn has a race problem. Films with people of color are often categorized by racial background, and sometimes it's used to play up the dramatics of the scene.

- Porn erases transgender people (especially nonbinary people and trans men) and demeans and misgenders them (especially trans women).

- Porn also reinforces heteronormativity in how it warps lesbian sex into "girl on girl" for the (assumed) straight, male viewer and defines "gay porn" only as sex between two men. "Gay porn" also only exists on sites completely separate from mainstream content.

- Porn has a male sexual supremacy problem and deems to dehumanize people who participate outside of the masculine gaze. In particular, pornography is known to oppress queer people with its rampant homophobia and heteronormativity.

- Porn doesn't explain consensual power dynamics. While the performers are consenting to a humiliation scene, we're not seeing that consent happen, so it can easily be misinterpreted. The scene often suggests that nonconsensual humiliation is OK to do.

- Porn has an aggressive effect on real-world sex. A 2013 Yale study found that long-term porn exposure makes men "animalify" women.

Porn's Impact on Real-World Sex

Porn is first and foremost a fantasy. It can be superhot and incredibly arousing, but porn has made a significant impact on how we engage in sex and communicate our sexual needs to our partners. In 2010, the University of Arkansas conducted a study that found that of the top fifty bestselling porn videos in the United States, 88 percent of them involved physical aggression. In 2015, Pornhub's Year in Review saw the search term "hard rough fuck" grow 454 percent. While porn is fantasy, the scenes we consume play a major role in how we see each other in real, non-porn intimacy—and porn has, in fact, been a catalyst for aggressive behavior in our culture. It can cause humans to develop body or performance insecurities, and make IRL sex seem unsatisfying and underwhelming; these things can negatively affect relationships when not addressed. Civilians see aggressive imagery with little to no consent context and believe that is the standard when it comes to sex. Plus, there is rampant mistreatment of porn talent that has gone unnoticed. Porn is enjoyable and useful, yes, but it can also be incredibly damaging when not viewed critically.

Is Porn Bad, Then?

Porn has its faults. Many faults. So, so many faults. But watching porn is a helpful tool in human arousal and can have a positive influence when we see it for what it is: a fantasy.

WHAT IF I LIKE SEX THE WAY THEY HAVE IT IN PORN?

So hot! That's super exciting and fun. But do your homework. Saying, "Fuck me like they do in porn," is a very vague sentence. What do you like? How do you like it? Is there anything you don't want to do or have done to you? And, does your partner want to be having this kind of sex? Is there after-care? If so, what is it? (See what aftercare might look like on page 222.) Masturbation, sex toys, and porn exploration will give you an incredibly good sense of what you're looking for, and you can communicate this to your partner(s). Have that conversation. Be open. Make room to discuss. Express clear consent if you both want to give it. If not, no is no.

WHAT IF I DON'T LIKE PORN?

Porn is not for everyone, and I absolutely get that. There will always be moments of sexual exploration that work for one person but don't work for another. And in the case of porn, there are plenty of pros and plenty of cons and all with dynamite arguments that can sway an opinion. So if you're not into porn, all good!

If you are, learn more about it! Sadly, porn stars face an incredible amount of stigma: They are often ostracized when seeking other employment, considered damaged or dirty, denied access to seeing their children, not given the same amount of dignity as others in public or private forums, and blamed if they do experience harm because the public believes they deserve it. This doesn't change as they get more experience, either—the porn industry is difficult for even the more seasoned performers. And this, I believe, stems from how we treat the erotic arts.

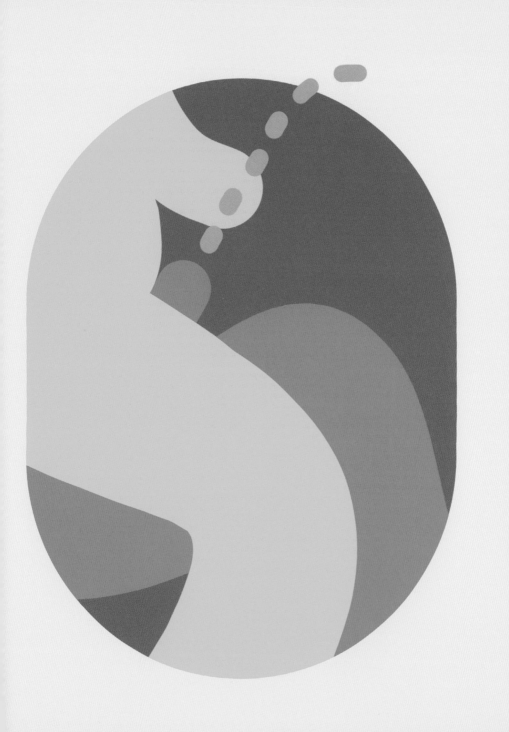

Personally, I see the value in pornography when looked at with a critical eye. Porn is both unreal and fully real at the same time. It's a fantasy and a movie set. It's a place for people to explore sexual interests and discover new arousal points, but also to confront unrealistic beauty standards and harmful sexual inclinations.

GOOD THINGS TO REMEMBER ABOUT LE PORNO

1| Porn is made to create arousal and to peek into the sexually explicit lives of others.

2| Porn is like making a movie. Yes, these are paid and hired actors. There is a call sheet, there is lighting, there is an editor, there are hair and makeup artists. Especially for mainstream pornography, making an erotic film is not so different from making a Hollywood film.

3| Intimacy coordinators are very real humans whose job is to keep talent safe on set when engaging in sexual activity. They work with actors and producers (who are also real humans) to create a safe environment and protect the talent.

4| Pursuing a career in the pornography business is difficult. It takes a lot of mental fortitude, the ability to make good decisions for your body, and the maturity to save money so it can last past retirement—which happens way sooner than you would think.

5| Viewers should treat porn stars as talent, not as commodities, and be selective with the porn they watch. That means consumers should pay for porn, research companies that hire diverse talent, look for companies run by women and people with marginalized identities (Black women, queer people, transgender people, people with disabilities), back companies that provide free STI testing to talent, and advocate for better terminology within porn so that talent is represented to the fullest extent of their identity.

Look, you're probably going to watch pornography. You might dabble in purchasing an erotic novel. You might even be turned on by a particularly hot almost-nude that you come across while scrolling on Instagram or Twitter. And that's fine! The erotic arts are alive and well because we are alive and well. As with everything else in this book, I want you to consider you. I want you to remember that a porn scene is not a reflection of real life. I want you to care about what you watch and the people performing for you. This kind of care feeds back into your decision-making, how you love yourself, and who you want to be.

HOW TO TALK ABOUT PORN WITH YOUR PARTNER Porn brings up a lot of feelings for people. It's important to take a moment and have a conversation with your partner about it. Maybe it's fine. Maybe it's a hot-button subject. No matter where you're both at, there are ways to have the conversation.

First, write down your feelings about porn. Now that you've gone through this chapter, maybe your feelings have changed. But what are they exactly? Do you like it? Do you hate it? Why? Does it make you feel insecure to know that your partner watches porn? Are there specific things that make you uncomfortable? Really understand what's in your brain before connecting with your partner.

Find neutral ground. It's not the best time to bring up porn preferences or watch porn together when you're in a fight, ya know? Take a walk and discuss it the same way you would when deciding what to have for dinner. Evoke that zero-pressure energy, babes!

Notice your insecurities and name them. You're allowed to feel a certain way. You're also allowed to not like things. But know why! The more you know about yourself, the more confident you'll feel in expressing your boundaries.

Discuss what you each most appreciate about porn. Discuss which types of scenes you like and don't like. Really get in there! Be your own expert and share that knowledge. There might be a subject you like, but your partner doesn't. All good! That will happen . . . and it's precisely why you want to keep this convo on neutral ground so that both of you can work from a practical place and not an emotional one.

If one partner doesn't want the other to watch porn without them, ask what is to be gained from that decision. Porn is a sensitive topic, so it's not unusual to feel odd when you know your partner is engaging in it without you. Instead of removing it altogether, have a conversation about your real sex life—bring it back to the two of you and what you love and what can be improved on.

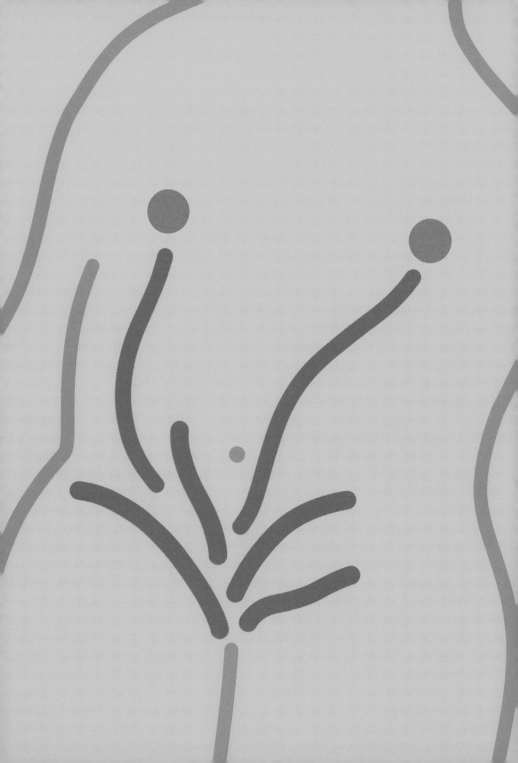

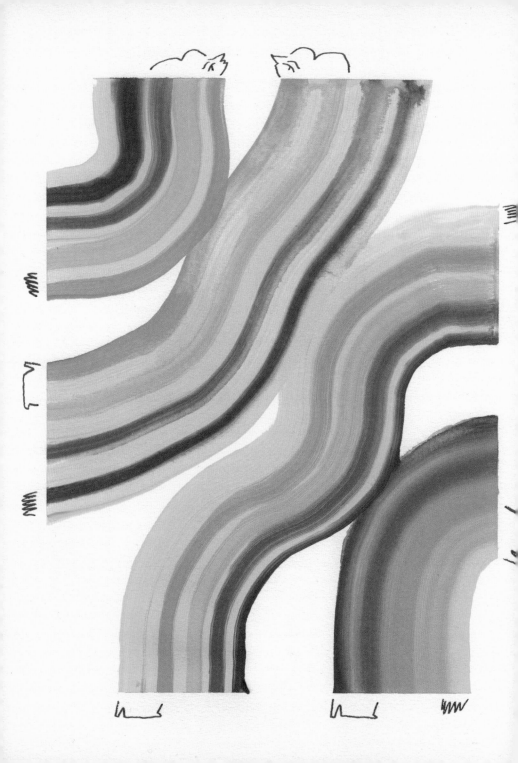

5

Partner

Play

You have come a long way from the start of this book—honoring your story, dating yourself, masturbating, identifying the perfect sex toy, and putting your pleasure at the top of the list each time.

Dang, you're living the most pleasurable life—keep up the excellent work!

Now, we're going to start adding lovers into the mix. This is your chance to expand on what you've learned about yourself and create a relationship—no matter its description. Exciting, right?!

Maybe you already have a partner; maybe you're not looking for one. Maybe you just want to have sexy sex sex with a person without any deeper attachments. Or maybe you want to explore what it means to date multiple people at the same time—awesome! However you want to approach dating and partnership is up to you. Let's get to it!

WHAT IS PARTNER PLAY?

Partner play is when two or more parties engage in emotional and sexual contact and connect over common interests. The relationship can be defined and redefined at any stage, but regardless of the label (or lack thereof), it requires all parties to listen and effectively communicate their needs, wants, and pleasures.

It's important to note that *partner play* is an umbrella term that can house many different types of relationships, which you can define for yourself. No need to stick to an arbitrary definition if it doesn't work for you! In fact, I encourage you to define your relationship in whatever way makes sense to you—don't worry too much about the label.

The good news is that there are many different types of relationships out there for you to explore if and when the time is right. Some are more casual while others are more committed, but all are a form of relationship that requires boundary setting, consent, and connection. See below for some relationship dynamics that might speak to your personality and interests—and if they don't, totally fine! Speak to your partner(s) about how you'd like to define your relationship and create your own definition.

COMMON RELATIONSHIP TYPES

- THE CASUAL RELATIONSHIP: This type of relationship is not formally defined—at least not yet—nor does it have a label, but it does involve a sexual relationship. While the casual relationship doesn't require a higher level of commitment, conversations around intimacy and personal boundaries should be had so that each person is on the same page.

- THE DATING RELATIONSHIP: This type of relationship is a step past casual, as there is active intention to get to know the other person/people and to create both an

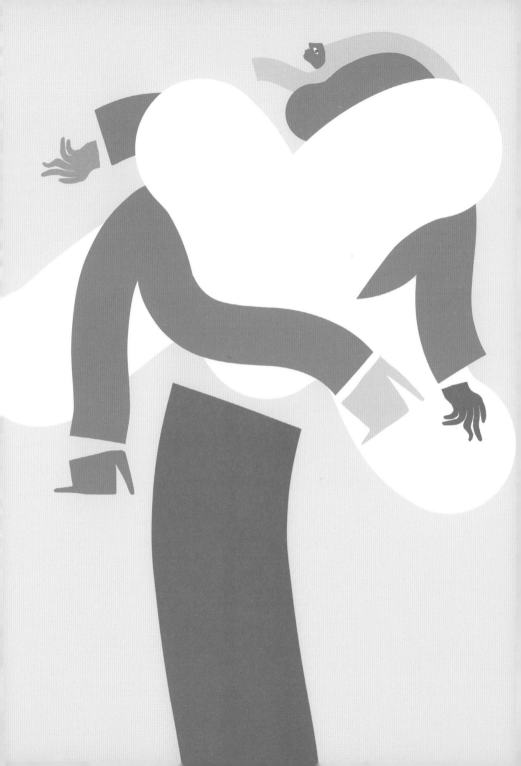

emotional and a sexual connection (if that is of interest to the parties involved).

- THE FRIENDS WITH BENEFITS RELATIONSHIP: This type of relationship blends together a natural friendship and sexual attraction without dating or committing to a more emotionally connected relationship. Note: These types of relationships are great but often require direct communication about what each person wants and how to move forward in the relationship.

- THE LONG-DISTANCE RELATIONSHIP: This type of relationship is an intimate bond between partners who are geographically separated from one another but still uphold boundaries by fostering trust and direct communication.

- THE MONOGAMOUS RELATIONSHIP: This type of relationship is when two humans are in a sexual partnership with one another and no one else.

- THE OPEN RELATIONSHIP: This type of relationship is an intimate connection that is sexually nonmonogamous. Some people in open relationships designate certain partners as their *primary* or their *person,* meaning that person is their main partner, while others stick to monikers such as *girlfriend, boyfriend, partner, spouse,* or *nesting partner* (meaning you live with them). Some nonmonogamous people use hierarchical language to describe their partners—for example, someone might have a primary or nesting partner, as well as a girl-friend whom they see casually and less frequently.

- THE PLATONIC RELATIONSHIP: This type of relationship is when two people love one another without a sexual component. Some people on the asexual spectrum may consider their romantic relationships platonic, but it depends on the person. This could be considered romantic or lean more toward friendship. Either way, it requires communication—just like every other relationship.

- THE PLAY PARTNERS: This type of relationship is when two or more people explore their kinks with each other. It's not a requirement for play partners to be in a sexual or romantic relationship (though they can be), but it does require trust and communication.

- THE POLYAMOROUS RELATIONSHIP: This type of relationship is when one person has open intimate and/or romantic relationships with more than one person at a time.

- THE THROUPLE RELATIONSHIP: This type of relationship involves three people who have consensually agreed to be in relationship together.

Every relationship has its own unique template. Make it your own.

To All the Lovers How do we feel about the word *lover*? I am kind of into it. But I do feel like I'm Rachel Dratch and Will Ferrell in that early-aughts *SNL* sketch: "The Love-ahs." I believe the reason I find it particularly uncomfortable to say in front of others is because I am then acknowledging my sex life or my alternative sex life to people who might not know me intimately—and I'm afraid of that judgment. Oh look! Something for me to work on! Sex stuff and body stuff and self-confidence . . . it's an ongoing lesson, reader.

Do You Need to Be Having Sex with a Partner to Have a Healthy Sex Life?

Not. At. All. Giving yourself time to explore your body and sexual interests solo is so incredibly valuable (see chapter 3) and, in turn, will make you more communicative if and when you decide to have sex, a relationship, a hookup, a masturbation session, a chill night where getting off isn't on your radar, or anything else. A healthy sex life is about communication, desire, and timing. Take your time and do what feels good to you.

As you find yourself exploring other people and different types of relationships, remember this: You have full control over your actions and the pleasure you would like to give and receive. Your superhot brain and body should come first. But

I'd also like to point out that putting your partner's sex needs first is also a massive component of being a great partner and improving your overall sex life! Some people even feel putting their partner's pleasure first is what gives them pleasure. So, like, put yourself first however that works for you.

Be kind to yourself, be caring about who you do and don't let into your life, be open to new possibilities, and be excited to share your pleasurable life with others.

WHAT ARE YOUR CORE SEX AND RELATIONSHIP VALUES?

The first step in understanding who you want to come into your pleasure circle is to identify your sex and relationship values. If we listen closely, our dates will tell us exactly who they are in our first meeting (or dating app message). You should never aim to change anyone, but simply to find whether they share your core values. Even if you're just looking for a hookup, it's still important to know whether your new potential lover is a decent person!

To answer this all-important question, respond to the following prompts. Write down your answers in a journal or notebook that you can easily reach for when deciding whether to go on that date or hook up with that person.

Your responses here should make it easy to answer the critical question: Will this potential partner contribute to your pleasurable life?

- List 3 to 5 of your most important personal values. Think back to your history, your pleasures, every moment you've had to reflect during the process of reading this book: What is most important to you in a relationship? Is it honesty? Excitement? Write 'em down! If you're already in a relationship, write down what you most value about your current relationship, as well as the ways you would like to connect more with your partner(s).

- List the 3 to 5 most important character attributes you want from a lover. These are words that would describe a prospective lover's personality. For example, you might write down: honest, responsive, kind, hardworking, energetic, brave, or creative. If you're already in a relationship, write what you most value about your current partner(s).

- List 3 to 5 sexual experiences you would like to have with a lover. Go on! Tell yourself all the hot things you want to do with your current boo or hypothetical new lover! It can be anything you want!

(As a reminder, this is a fun list for you, but consent is 100 percent needed in order to move forward with any of these actions.)

- List 3 to 5 ways you want to feel around this new lover or current relationship and why. For example, you might write that you want to feel safe with them, as safety is something you value after a past experience made you feel unsafe. This can be anything and for any reason—you just have to be honest!

Rethink the First Date

Getting to know someone can be exciting, exhausting, and a little bit tiptoe-y as you both try to navigate each other's personality. The one thing we are taught by every representation of dating is that you shouldn't ask tough questions on the first date lest you scare off your partner. I say to hell with that.

Of course, be respectful. But dating is like an interview for a prospective candidate: You have to ask the questions in order to see whether you and they are aligned. Yes, please, ask about who they are, their pronouns, where they grew up, and whether they have any cool tattoos. But also feel free to dig a little deeper. Ask for what you want. Ask for it ASAP from your dates and refuse to be shy about it. Keep in mind that this person doesn't have to be a 100 percent perfect match, but they do need to exemplify the sex and relationship values that you identify with. (Take a peek at your values list to remind yourself of exactly who you are and what you believe in.) Here are some questions you may want to ask.

STRAIGHT-TO-THE-POINT FIRST-DATE QUESTIONS

- "What is your stance on safer sex?"

It is a fair question to anyone who is interested in being naked with you.

- "Tell me about the people—women, men, nonbinary—in your life."

This is not a question to decipher whether any exes are still in the picture—this is about understanding how they speak about others and whether it's respectful.

- "What is a long-term life goal that you have for yourself?"

You're not out here showing bank account receipts or anything like that. You're looking at their ambition and whether it matches yours.

DOES THIS PERSON/DATE/ACTIVITY
ALIGN WITH MY VALUES?

If you're not sure whether a certain sexual interaction or date is worth your time, ask yourself the following questions and really consider whether and how your responses reflect your core values:

- What do I need right now? Do I need physical affection? Or do I need to sleep? Do I need to eat? Do I need to cry? Will this interaction take away from those basic needs?

- Is this person respectful of others? What do I know about this person?

- Will I have to spend money for dinner or drinks before even getting to know this person? Am I willing to do that?

- Does this require me to travel? If so, am I up for that?

- How do I feel when I talk to this person? Have they said anything that I thought was a red flag but dismissed because I was aroused and wanted things to work out?

COMMUNICATION IS KEY

Yes, no, maybe so—communication is a deeply important part of the partner play experience. In fact, throughout all your current and future relationships, whether they are romantic, casual, or platonic, good communication is vital. It is the key to effective and long-term relationships with others as well as with yourself.

Mind you, it takes a lot of effort to be aware of your own wants and needs, let alone navigating those of another person. So far in this book, you have gotten really, really good at communicating with yourself about what you want and need, but how does that translate to communicating with another person who is interested in getting naked with you? How do you communicate your needs while also meeting theirs? And what happens if you disagree about something?

Oh no! A dreaded disagreement! I hate to break it to you, but no matter how simpatico you and your new lover are, there will always be something you don't agree on and need to work through. This is why excellent communication skills are important. While Disney movies, rom-coms, and the entirety of the Hallmark Channel will try to convince you that there is only one true, uncomplicated, no-work-to-be-had love out there for everyone, I will stand in defiance and tell you that that is simply false. No matter how much you gel with another person, you will, at some point, need to communicate about uncomfortable, complicated, or sticky issues in order to feel fully seen and to explore new, exciting possibilities with your lover. Shoving those feelings down shuts us off to other people and makes it extremely difficult to find pleasure, babes.

What Is Your Communication Style?

Depending on our history, upbringing, and the societal gender expectations we were taught, we all have a different way of communicating. The most common communication styles are passive, aggressive, passive-aggressive, manipulative, and assertive.

Knowing our own communication style as well as that of our partner(s) allows us to be effective communicators and find common ground with others. (This is true outside of intimate relationships too, say at a work meeting or a holiday party with difficult family members.) Most of us have various communication styles with one primary style that takes charge. Which one are you? Read the following descriptions and note which kind of communicator you are. When these styles become present in a conversation, bring awareness to it, and reconsider how to continue the discussion.

- PASSIVE: This person is afraid to say no, refuses to create conflict, and often gives in to what others want. There is often underlying frustration or resentment associated with this communication style, as this person's

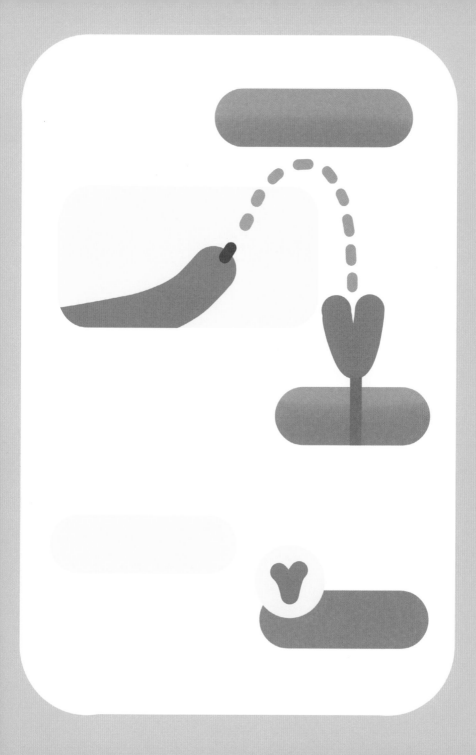

needs are often not being met. If this is you, consider finding ways to be more vocal about your opinions and what you need. Being an effective communicator doesn't mean you have to be demanding—it means you have to speak up.

- AGGRESSIVE: This person isn't afraid of being hostile or rude to get their way. In fact, they're typically insensitive to other people's feelings in order to control the situation—and that will cause others to feel disrespected and to push away. If this is you, consider asking for other people's opinions and taking a moment to explore whether a situation requires the power of an aggressive leader or a bit of compassion. Sure, you might have the best idea, but not everyone will stand by you if they don't feel heard.

- PASSIVE-AGGRESSIVE: This person will tell others what they want to hear to avoid conflict but won't follow through on the agreed-upon plan. This will leave others confused, frustrated, and resentful when you don't meet the desired expectations. If this is you, try to be up front with how you're feeling and provide clear and actionable goals that you will commit to so others know they are being heard.

- MANIPULATIVE: This person will attempt to get their way by making others feel guilty, and will often take the role of the victim so others will assume responsibility for taking care of this person's needs. If this feels like your communication style, try to be more mindful of your own actions and reactions. That way, you can start to see others' reactions as valid and begin to hold space for their feelings.

- ASSERTIVE: This person is direct and honest about their needs and wants, while taking responsibility for themselves and also being respectful of others. This person is an effective listener and finds ways to stand up for their interests without downplaying the feelings of others.

Helpful Communication Techniques

I'd love to tell you that when two people care about each other, all of their communication is easy and clear. But this isn't true. My human experience is going to be different from yours, which will be different from anyone else's. It's important to recognize this very human dilemma and embrace effective communication techniques to be on the same page with your partner.

- TRY THE GIBBERISH TECHNIQUE. If neither of you is getting your point across, or if someone is starting to get frustrated in the process, a really good trick is to drop all language for 30 seconds and speak to each other

in gibberish! Yeah, it's silly and odd and fun and it
de-escalates the conversation so that you and your
partner (or lover or friend or parent) can continue
without any animosity.

- USE SAFE WORDS WHEN HAVING A DISCUSSION—especially one
  on a sensitive topic—so that either party can ease any
  tension if the conversation starts to become frustrating or murky. (More on safe words on page 205.)

- LEARN TO SPEAK WITHOUT FEAR, HESITATION, OR WORRY by recognizing your voice patterns when speaking about
  inconsequential topics. For example, asking your
  partner what they want to eat for dinner could be less
  stressful than asking a partner to watch porn and
  masturbate together, depending on your dynamic.
  Notice how calm you sound in different, less weighted
  scenarios and bring that into how you communicate
  on more sensitive topics.

- DROP SOMETHING! No, really! Verbal communication is
  not always available. Create a nonverbal system with
  your partner by dropping unbreakable objects when
  you need to stop a conversation or slow down. Think:
  scarf or pillow. Or, in a sexual context, use a light-up
  toy to communicate that you need a check-in if you're
  struggling to speak up. Even in the dark, the light from

the toy will draw attention, and even if you are tied up, you can still drop the toy.

You Can Always Say No

Something to consider in the communication process: All of us deserve to be heard, but not everything deserves a yes. Let's say you're speaking to your play partner about different sex acts that you both want to perform on each other, and your play partner would like you to do something you're uncomfortable with. No matter how you feel, you should make space for what the other person is saying so there can be effective communication throughout the relationship, but you're allowed to disagree and say no to what is being asked of you.

In other words, communication doesn't automatically mean saying yes. This, friends, is the tenet of consent.

Prioritizing Your Pleasure When I think of living a pleasurable life, I think of a rom-com divorcée who squeezes fresh orange juice every day and brings croissants in a basket wherever she goes. She, obviously, has a garden and only wears cream-colored clothes; she spends hours reading from a bench in the park, casually gazing up to watch the surrounding action. This divorcée has many lovers—some more serious than others. They come to her place—she never goes to theirs—and she takes a long bath before sex so she can feel relaxed and present in her body. She lives by her own rules, which are guided by her pleasures.

This is my ideal of a pleasurable life, and I encourage you to envision yours. No matter what it looks like for you, one of the first steps we can all take to get there is to practice saying no. Saying no can be incredibly difficult: Society has taught some of us to be good, to service others, to be helpful—all of which means saying yes. But saying yes to everything and everyone else means less time for the things you actually care about. We're in the twenty-first century. It's time to prioritize yourself and the things you care about so that you too can have multiple lovers, wear cream-colored clothing, and eat croissants every day without a care in the world.

What Is Consent?

Consent occurs when one person voluntarily agrees to the proposal or desires of another. Consent is a requirement for sexual intimacy of any kind. A few notes on consent:

- CONSENT IS SINGULAR. Just because you give someone consent to kiss you doesn't mean they have the right to take off your clothes. Consent isn't a package deal.

- CONSENT TODAY DOESN'T MEAN CONSENT TOMORROW. Just because you consented in the past doesn't mean that consent is open for any future participation.

- YOU CAN CHANGE YOUR MIND AT ANY TIME. Yes, this means that you can be in the middle of sexual activity or even a date and stop the entire thing if you want.

- INCAPACITATED CONSENT IS NOT CONSENT. If you or another party is not in their right state of mind (whether that is from emotional duress or alcohol or drug consumption), they are not able to make the proper judgment call required to say yes or no.

- BE CLEAR HOW YOU CONSENT. Not everyone has the ability to use verbal cues to initiate consent—but we also shouldn't assume that smiling means consent. Writing consent down on a piece of paper, using sign language with another party that definitively understands, or even showing different flash card colors or digital representations of red (no) and green (yes) are all viable ways to make consent known. Before you engage in any kind of sexual act, decide how you will give consent, particularly if verbal consent is not an option. Clarity will keep our hearts, minds, and bodies safe and excited to play!

The best way to avoid being misunderstood or misunderstanding your partner is to regularly check in with them about how they are feeling. Do their actions and interests match yours? Communication is key not only to having a hot sex life, but also to the safety and care of others.

A no is a no is a no. Saying no to something you don't want to do is simultaneously saying yes to the person you are and the boundaries you hold. Be proud of that.

THE YES/NO/MAYBE LIST

Let's say you have a new romantic partner whom you want to get to know on a more sexual level. Sure, you can have dinner and figure it all out on the way to the bedroom—or you can really build anticipation and communication at the same time with a little game called the Yes/No/Maybe List.

Before meeting up to discuss what you're both interested in, each person should go through a list of sex acts separately and decide whether they are yes, interested; no, not interested; or maybe interested; and whether or not they would like to give or receive the acts they mark as a yes. This list can either come from the internet (there are a lot of lists out there from reputable sources) or use the one provided. Or make your own!

Why separately? Well, it's pretty hot to come to the table with all your yeses and see what you both put down. Imagine you and your new boo grabbing a coffee at an outdoor cafe, and sipping your espresso while the sexual tension builds and builds and builds. So hot. But also, creating the list separately allows for each person to be honest about their hard yeses and nos without being influenced by, or wanting to please, the other person. This list is about you, and the fun comes in where you both overlap.

This also gives you a chance to establish your hard nos—that is, the acts that you will not be participating in under any circumstances. Nos don't require any more explanation other than you're just not into them. Maybes are there for you both to discuss, explore, and become more educated about; perhaps you'll even attend a workshop on the topic. And mutual yeses are your common ground where you both can play—of course, with consent.

This is a fun exercise to repeat over time because you can see what you've enjoyed, lost interest in, or become open to from year to year. Plus, it's a great way to have a conversation with your sex partners about what you want!

Not sure where to start? Start here! See the following list of very fun sex acts. Write down yes, no, or maybe next to each act and, where applicable, whether you want to give or receive (or both) with your partner. Get to know yourself with some of these fun, sexy options below. If there is something here that interests you, consider learning about it by taking a class. Ask yourself: Where on the body would I like to try this, how soft, how hard, what kind of impact, what is the possible danger? Make sure you're aware of the risks involved before going forward.

- Anal fingering
- Anal intercourse
- Anal massage
- Anal penetration
- Biting
- Blindfolding
- Bondage
- Breast play
- Dry humping
- Ejaculating in a partner's body
- Ejaculating on a partner's body
- Hand or digit sex (i.e., hand job or fingering)
- Hickeys/visible marks
- Holding hands
- Hugging
- Impact play
- Kissing
- Massage
- Masturbating next to or in front of your partner(s)
- Nipple play
- Open mouth kissing
- Oral sex to penis
- Oral sex to strap-on
- Oral sex to vulva
- Pinching
- Restricting movements
- Role-playing
- Rope play
- Scratching
- Slapping
- Solo masturbation
- Spanking
- Strap-on play
- Tickling
- Tribadism (a.k.a. scissoring)
- Using food items as a part of sex
- Using sex toys on a partner
- Using sex toys with a partner
- Vaginal intercourse
- Wearing clothes of the opposite gender
- Wrestling or "play fighting"

To make space or hold space for someone
is to be physically, mentally, and
emotionally present for that person.

How to Communicate and Find Intimacy at a Distance

Physical distance always makes things really difficult, even when all parties are trying their best to maintain an open and intimate relationship. Long-distance relationships are not impossible, but they do require some work. Creating a yes/no/maybe list when you're not in the same place to act out all your fantasies might not be an option—or perhaps you have to rethink what that list looks like. However, there are other cool ways to have some erotic fun when you're a phone call or text away.

- EROTICA BOOK CLUB. Have a little fun by choosing a sexy book to read each month. Set up a time to chat about it—or even video chat and act out a scene or two! Highlight sections that you'd be interested in recreating and send them to your partner when they need a sexy pick-me-up!

- APP-BASED SEX TOYS. There are sex toys that can be operated with a touch from any smartphone. (Technology is amazing, isn't it?!) Do a little research and find the right toy for you; then, give your partner control for a night.

- DIGITAL ROLE-PLAY. Maybe you "accidentally called the wrong number," but find yourself speaking to a very attractive-sounding person and need to see where it takes you!

- SEXTING. The thrill of having a sexy message pop up on your phone's home screen will send a sexually charged shock through your system.

- VIDEO STRIPTEASE. The device in our pockets is a gateway to literally having a video conversation with another human. We are in the future! And in this future, it's superhot to act out a whole routine that makes you feel both good and horny.

- SEXY SNAIL MAIL. Set up your camera, snap some boudoir photos, and send them to your lover with a handwritten message listing all the hot ways you want them to touch you.

LOVERS AND LIMITS

Whenever I get asked what my "type" is, I always say that my type is someone who sees it as a priority to keep my heart, my mind, and my body safe. Honestly! There is something really arousing about connecting with another levelheaded adult who actually cares about me and my pleasures. (For example, I'm 100 percent sure Zac Efron would prioritize me and honor my boundaries.)

There is so much more to sex than genitalia and orgasms. There is a whole world out there to explore: tenderness, roughness, playing with power, creating a full scene around spanking (exciting!), kink (sexual activity that falls outside of what popular society considers conventional sexual interactions), and so much more. When exploring new sexual activities, trust is deeply important. Remember that your limits always deserve to be honored. In this section, we'll talk about sexual limits, how to create a safe environment, feelings of jealousy, and more. Before we get started, here are some good terms to learn and use as we start to talk about trust, limits, and our lovers:

- TOP/TOPPING: The partner who performs.

- BOTTOM/BOTTOMING: The partner who receives.

- SUB/SUBMISSIVE/SUBMISSION: The partner who is being controlled or the act of being controlled.

- DOM/DOMINANT/DOMINANCE: The partner who is controlling or the act of controlling another person.

- SCENE: The scenario in which all the sexual or erotic activity is occurring.

- PLAY: The actions/activities inside the scene.

- BOUNDARY/LIMIT: The invisible barrier that cannot be crossed by anyone.

(For more sexy, must-know terms, take a look at the glossary on page 232.)

Sexual Limits

HOW DO I TALK ABOUT MY SEXUAL LIMITATIONS WITH A POTENTIAL OR CURRENT PARTNER?

Any conversation that requires one person to speak about a vulnerable topic can definitely cause nervousness, *but this shouldn't be a stressful conversation*! In fact, it should be a positive discussion and an opportunity to stand up for what you need in order to feel pleasure.

Let's say you really need to refrain from being on your knees at any point during sexual activity. It hurts even with a pillow! Set some time aside to have that conversation and talk about it the way you would when trying to figure out what to watch on Netflix (see Helpful Communication Techniques on page 193). If it still makes you nervous, practice having the conversation with yourself and saying what you'd like to say:

"Babe, I love when we do _____, but dang, it really hurts my knees. Maybe we can figure out a different solution to that position?"

Clear, simple, understandable. And here is the really creative part: We often look at our physical limitations as this end-of-the-road, can't-do-that-ever-again situation. But really, it gives you and your partner the opportunity to explore other positions and other moves.

Can't be on your knees? All good! What if you laid on your back? What if you invested in some sex furniture that would help you ease into a better position? Explore all the opportunities to make this limitation into a positive.

LIMITATIONS ARE AN OPPORTUNITY

We all have something that make sex and intimacy a little more difficult, and this can be super frustrating . . . but it doesn't have to be! With every limitation comes an opportunity to expand and evolve our sexual horizons.

- Lack hand dexterity? . . . Try a thigh harness! It can hold a dildo in place on your thigh and is also great for mobility.

- Need to be seated? . . . Consider a swing.

- Can't rest weight on joints? . . . Plush sex furniture or pillows will do the trick!

- Standing isn't an option? . . . Lie down!

Safe Words

Since we're speaking about limits and boundaries, this would be a good time to bring up safe words. When thinking about your limitations and how to have the utmost pleasure from your partnered sexual experiences, safe words should be a central part of the discussion.

A safe word is a singular word or a series of words, signals, or codes used to communicate a person's physical or emotional state. Typically, these sets of words exist outside of "yes" or "no" or even "I like that" and "I don't like that," as those could be misconstrued as part of the fantasy or scene you and your partner have built for yourselves.

Typically, safe words are used during sex, scenes, or any kind of sexual play to indicate that a boundary is being crossed or is coming close to being crossed. At that point, the giver of the stimulation should stop all play and remove their partner from any restrictive position.

HOW DO I PICK A SAFE WORD?

Safe words are agreed upon by all people in the scene or sexual play. They can really be anything. I quite enjoy "Stoplight." *Red* means stop, *yellow* means slow down, and *green* means yes, yes, keep going! It is also useful to use *blue* within the stoplight method to signify to a partner that you are feeling triggered. But it really all depends on the people involved and how the safe words are communicated.

WHEN CAN A SAFE WORD BE USED?

Anytime! Look, if you're uncomfortable, you should 100 percent let your partner know. Self-love, body love, and a healthy sex life are all about making sure you're having a good time and honoring your boundaries.

DOES CALLING A SAFE WORD MEAN THAT THE GIVER HAS DONE SOMETHING WRONG?

In short, no, not necessarily. It's possible that the giver in this scenario forgot about the specific boundary or a new boundary came up for the receiver in the middle of the play. All this requires is a check-in and re-communication of the boundaries.

ARE SAFE WORDS ONLY FOR SEX?

Nope! In fact, safe words are an excellent way to communicate your feelings to a partner when having a heated discussion. Sometimes, a conversation is best put on hold and resumed later, when feelings are not running so high. Using a safe word when it starts to get argumentative can help de-escalate the situation and put things into perspective.

EXCELLENT SAFE WORDS TO USE

Feel free to create your own or use multiple words to mean different exclamations. Be clear and simple when choosing safe words so everyone understands!

CATEGORIES

- Stoplight (see facing page)

- Fruits (for example, *peach* means yes but *dragon fruit* means no)

- US presidents (for example, *Kennedy* means yes, *Nixon* means no)

HARD NOS

- Cinnamon

- Kiefer Sutherland (this is mine, but I'll let you borrow it)

- Calculator

- Submarine

- Fake news

- Cosmopolitan

- Envelope

- Canterbury

- Macintosh

WHAT IF I LIKE IT ROUGH? SHOULD I BE EMBARRASSED TO ASK FOR THAT?

Not at all, my sexy sex reader. It's good to know where you fall in the sexual play arena. Ask yourself what you mean by "rough." Can you verbally describe it? Are there visual references that you can use? Because your idea of rough might exist outside of your partner's boundaries or they might have a completely different definition or understanding of what "rough" is. Having specifics in mind when you communicate with your partner will help. Don't just say, "I like it rough." Explain your thinking.

For this activity, consider how you would explain your sexual interests to your partner(s). See the following prompts for how to strike up that conversation. Feel free to add your own! Once you have your ideal list, practice saying them to yourself so it becomes part of the norm in your brain and stops feeling embarrassing or shameful to ask.

"I love it when I feel your

_____ in/on my_____."
BODY PART   BODY PART

"Make my _____ _____."
           BODY PART   VERB

"Give your _____ to me."
           BODY PART

"I would love it if we could

try _____."
    SEX ACT

"How would you feel about

_____ my _____?"
VERBING   BODY PART

"Want to try _____ my/your

_____?" VERBING
BODY PART

"Are you into _____ tonight?"
         SEX ACT

NOTE: If you don't like it rough, that's also really OK! If a partner is going a little too fast or hard in any way, you can always draw from your safe words, consider a new position, take a break, or stop completely. It's your body. You decide how you want to experience pleasure.

What About Jealousy?

Ah yes, jealousy. 'Tis a thing that we all need to be aware of. Interestingly enough, jealousy has very little to do with our partner's actions. Often, it comes from our own insecurities and bouts of low self-esteem, especially if we have chosen to see multiple people or engage in an open relationship with clear boundaries. This is where our trust and limits will be challenged, and we might feel the pressure to bend our needs to benefit the other person. But you're both doing this together, and together all of your needs can be met. Consider these tips on staying focused and using that jealous energy for good:

- If there is another person in your partner's life that is well within the boundaries of the relationship, consider them an ally. This doesn't mean you need to be in contact with them if you're not up for it, but there is a reason your partner cares for them and you should hold them in your heart with the same respect your partner does.

- There is a lot of good that can come from having space and interacting with different people who have different perspectives. While this is true in monogamous relationships, it is particularly applicable and helpful to internalize if you're in an open relationship. Take solace in the fact that you and your partner are learning how to be great partners and communicators from each other and from other people—double the learning!

- If your partner has crossed a boundary with you by seeing another person, bring it up. You're not in the business of hiding your feelings! Have a conversation about where the partnership should go and/or what needs to be rebuilt.

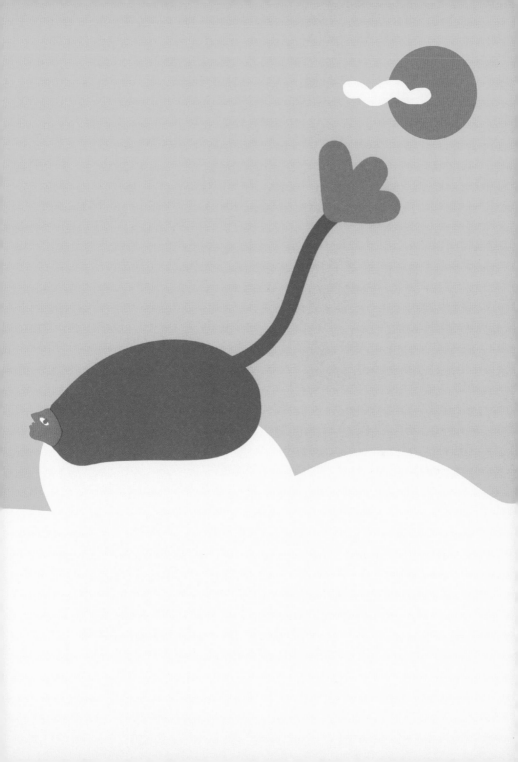

- Remember, feelings aren't facts. Feelings, especially jealous feelings, can often spiral out of control. Take a moment to remember what is factually true and what is not.

How to Open Up a Closed Relationship

All this jealousy talk might have you wondering how a couple can open up their relationship the right way. Well, first, there isn't a right way. There is a way and there will be bumps along that path, but trust, good communication, and clear boundaries will allow each person to have their needs met respectfully. But how to do it?

- BE HONEST WITH YOURSELF. What is the need and why? Find the truth in your heart and analyze it straight on. For example, let's say you have a fantasy that requires anonymity. All good! Get into the crumbs of this desire and be open to this vulnerability.

- COME TO THE CONVERSATION WITH GOOD INTENTIONS. Find time when both parties are in a neutral state. Don't spring this idea on someone right in the middle of a disagreement or when you're lying in bed about to fall asleep. Don't send them a text. Set up time to check in with your partner in a common area like a restaurant or a museum. If you're looking to have a more private conversation, consider a neutral space so each person feels comfortable to speak.

- GIVE THEM TIME TO PROCESS. You can't expect anyone to give an answer right away. They might not be into it. They might have an emotional reaction. They might be more interested in it than you are! All are valid. Think of it as a business decision. You need to weigh the pros and cons and criteria before signing on the dotted line.

- DO IT TOGETHER. You don't have to be on each other's dating apps, but have some fun with it! Swipe for the other person, become experts on the subject of openness, take classes, sign up for workshops, go to couple's therapy, create date nights and special time for just each other. Openness isn't something to shy away from with your partner. You're in this together!

- SET BOUNDARIES. This goes for emotional, sexual, and physical boundaries. An emotional boundary means considering the who and why behind each partner's dates. For example, is it OK if your partner dates an ex or someone in your friend circle? Sexual boundaries are around the sex acts that you're not OK with your partner engaging in. For example, are you comfortable with oral sex but not with penetrative sex? What are the boundaries around safer sex? (Note: All

sex involves some level of risk even if it is emotional
rather than physical.) A physical boundary is about
location and the distance between partners. For
example, do these dates happen at your shared home
or at the other person's home? Do either of you want
to know about the dates and the details of what went
down? All the nitty-grittiness should be considered!
Maybe even write them down.

- NOTE HOW THIS INFORMATION IS TO BE DISCUSSED. This is a great
time to bring in safe words! Yes, most of the time safe
words are there to vocalize that you want to stop. In
this case, you can use them to introduce information
and give your partner the chance to make time for the
discussion. Let's say you want to inform your partner that you'd like to go on a date on Thursday. Consider bringing it up in a calm way and during a quiet
moment in the day, and use a safe word to preface the
convo. For example: "Hi, babe! I'd love to talk with you
about plans with Watermelon when you have a free
moment." It's possible they're busy or stressed or can't
talk right then, and this approach gives your partner
the opportunity to discuss the situation when they
feel comfortable.

- CREATE CHECK-INS. It's possible things might not go as
planned the first time around. That's OK! Note the

parts of the experience that weren't so great and discuss them at the next check-in with your partner. These can be once a week, once a month, or every other month just to chat about openness and how it's benefiting the relationship. Again, find your honesty and let it guide you.

Kink and Lovers

As noted prior, *kink* is defined as sexual activity that falls outside of what popular society considers conventional sexual interactions. It's often a heightened form of play that can involve role-playing, BDSM (bondage, discipline, dominance, submission, sadism, switching, and masochism), power exchange, impact on the body, pain, or even humiliation.

Kink is an excellent way to develop more trust and connection with your partner(s). When partaking in kink, each person needs to understand and consent to the physical and emotional risks involved. Also, they need to be aware of their partner's boundaries, preferences, health issues, past trauma, triggers to avoid, and safe words. It's vital to have a discussion around what both people are consenting to performing on the other person and on themselves. Honestly, it should be like one big musical theater production where everyone knows their cue all the way to the closing number and the wrap party.

BUT IS IT WEIRD?

Not at all! Kink is a perfectly healthy way to express your sexual desires or even your inner emotions—and actual sex doesn't even need to be involved if you don't want it to be. Think of kink as an erotic way to explore different expressions of yourself. As far as limits go, kink is an excellent way to build trust with your partner and to honor those boundaries with creative (and sexy) workarounds.

HOW DO I BRING IT UP TO A PARTNER?

There are many different ways to have that conversation with a person you trust or want to build trust with, but first consider how you feel. Are you excited? Awesome! Consider setting up a date with your lover to discuss new ways to be more intimate in bed. Maybe send them a sexy calendar invite with the expectation of dinner and exploration.

If you're nervous, say so! It's perfectly OK to come from a place of vulnerability. Also, do some research—but leave a little for you and your partner to do together. If you have any specific ideas, talk about them! In this book, you have spent many an activity considering the pleasure you want; this is an awesome chance to put that into action.

Not everyone is going to positively react to this conversation— and that's OK! This topic can bring up a lot of shame, and not everyone has done the personal work to understand why. Maybe it's embarrassment, maybe it's fear of looking silly, maybe there is a past trauma they haven't considered yet. Make sure your partner is enthusiastically consenting to exploration, and respect how they are feeling. (Remember, if the conversation gets a little too heated, anyone can pull a safe word to pause and continue the conversation at another time.)

A Few Types of Kink

Kink is a sexual category for anyone to explore on their own and in their own time—especially considering how much of kink can really tap into deeper emotions. The following options show how to incorporate some of the more popular (or well-known) kink scenes into your pleasure world.

- AGE PLAY is a type of role-playing in which we consensually act or treat others as if they were a different age, whether in a sexual or a nonsexual context. Assuming it is performed between two consenting adults of legal age, age play is a great way to play out a teacher/ student fantasy or reimagine an experience from a different perspective.

- BDSM is a multitude of erotic practices involving bondage, discipline, dominance, submission, sadism, switching, and masochism. BDSM can include spanking, tying up a partner, receiving or giving different forms of pain, or using handcuffs, blindfolds, whips, or paddles. Sexual release may not even be necessary for some scenes, as the core of BDSM is role-playing and creating characters who act out interpersonal dynamics.

- FETISH refers to an attraction to an inanimate object, such as lingerie, or body parts, such as feet.

- IMPACT PLAY is a practice in which one person is consensually struck by another person for erotic gratification. Have you ever wanted to try spanking or slapping? Are you turned on by the idea of being punished? Impact play can heighten pleasure and create a fun power dynamic between parties.

- KINK TOYS include the aforementioned paddle, whip, handcuffs, and blindfolds. Also in this category are hoods, collars, ball gags, nipple clamps, floggers, and restraints. There is something so fun and delicious about being outfitted with all the items you need to create a rockin' good erotic night. Kink toys are an amazing addition to anyone's sex drawer, just as long as they're used with consent.

- POWER DYNAMICS is the exchange of power between people and can be a fun element in consensual role-playing. If you're usually more dominant in the bedroom, try playing the more submissive role, or vice versa. There is a lot to learn in seeing things from the other side.

- ROLE-PLAYING is acting out a scene or performing as a character during an erotic or sexual experience. It can be such fun to embody another person, making the choices that they would make, and maybe even engaging in some new sexual play that they like. I always think about drag queen transformations when it comes to role-play—the face changes, the walk changes, and the mannerisms change.

- SENSATION PLAY employs objects and substances to stimulate the body's neuroreceptors for sensual effect. This can be related to temperature or other sensations. For example, an ice cube on the nipple, dripping body-safe hot wax, or even lightly dragging flower petals and a thorny stem across your partner's chest can be incredibly erotic—use a blindfold for a more heightened effect.

- VOYEURISM is the sexual pleasure derived from watching others when they are naked or partaking in sexual activity. This can be as simple as letting your partner "catch" you showering, watching them masturbate, or inviting other play partners over to peek at your or their fun—consensually, of course.

ROLE-PLAY SCENARIOS Playing a completely different person allows you to test new circumstances that you may be too embarrassed or self-conscious to do as yourself. You can explore power in a way that might not come naturally in your day-to-day life. Ever want to take control? Give it up? Surrender yourself to what comes next? Role-play allows you to do so safely. Maybe there is something new to explore as the boss or assistant or nurse or patient—you get the idea. Try out some of the following options or create a list of your own to explore!

- THE STRANGER: Arrange to meet at a new location with completely different names and backstories. See where the night takes you!

- THE BUTLER: Oh wow, the butler is looking superhot today! Set up a scenario where one person is in service to the other, and play out the evening in character!

- THE MASSEUSE: There is nothing better than pampering yourself with a nice massage by someone who knows how to use their hands!

- THE PIZZA DELIVERY PERSON: A classic, but definitely worth the experience. You open the door to your pizza delivery, but oh gosh . . . you don't have any money! How will you pay?!

- THE ARTIST: You're there to be sketched naked by a hot artist when you start to get aroused. What do you do?

SPANKING 101

When we talk about impact play or BDSM, spanking tends to be the first item on that checklist. And while popular culture would have us believe that we simply haul off and hit another person in the name of kink (no), there are some safety precautions to take before spanking someone or being spanked for the first time!

- Talk to each other: Who is the giver, who is the receiver, what will you be using, where do you want to strike, and does that feel good to all parties?

- Be aware of where you can strike: It's always a good rule to stay within fleshy areas of the body such as the butt, thighs, and chest. Avoid the kidney area (sides), neck, joints, tailbone, hips, and spine.

- Use a safe word: Pick anything you'd like that will symbolize stop and slow down. The red, yellow, green language is a great option!

- Get turned on: Watch porn, make out, touch each other, touch yourself! The body reacts better to pain when aroused.

- Start slow: Do a few little taps to start.

- Use a scale of 1 to 10: As the spanker ramps up the force behind each spank, they ask the receiver what level of pain they are at and where their limit is.

- Know the types of spanks: Not every spank is a slap to the ass. Some spanks can be done with the fist or the tips of your fingers. Some can be a slap and an immediate release. Or you can alternate. Mix both stinging and thudding spanks into your play.

- Rub the area: It can really hurt to get spanked, tops! Giving a nice rub to the area afterward can keep an ongoing connection with your bottom as you both reach your goals.

- Communicate: You don't have to ask, "Hey, are you OK?" You can use your safe words in a sexy way: "You like getting spanked, don't you? Does this feel like a green, you (fill in sexy, dirty pet name here)?"

- Feel the sensations: Now that the blood is drawn to the surface of the skin, try some light scratching or rubbing an ice cube on the area for other sensations.

- Be mindful of the time: There will be a natural start and end to the play as the spanking ramps up, but a great way to track yourself is by playing music! Give yourself the length of three songs, check in, and see if you both want to continue.

- Don't forget the aftercare: Impact play allows the bottom to experience a unique emotional release while simultaneously enduring pain. Keep water and snacks available for your bottom. Listen to them if they need to lie down or be held or have some alone time. Aftercare is a crucial part of all kink play!

What Can Aftercare Look Like?

Aftercare is typically the attention the top gives to a bottoming partner at the end of a scene. Why do this? Well, because any scene, whether it's sexy or kinky or both, can spike endorphins and adrenaline depending on what is taking place, and this can cause people to feel lightheaded, emotional, deeply exhausted, or dizzy. Sometimes this is referred to as subspace (an emotional and psychological out-of-body experience in reaction to the adrenaline and endorphins). Because it's so sudden, it's important to have a system of aftercare in place if or when subspace is experienced.

Prior to the play, all partners need to negotiate and come to a firm agreement of what the aftercare will look like and when it will happen. Tops, bottoms, dominants, submissives, and switches all need aftercare, so it's important to discuss, map out, and agree to what that will look like when ending a scene.

AFTERCARE CAN LOOK LIKE:

- Giving space

- Cuddling

- Providing food and water

- Giving a light massage

- Holding a partner

- Running your partner a bath

PLEASURABLE PARTNER PLAY

No matter what you and your partner or multiple partners do in bed (or in the kitchen, living room, etc.), it should come from a place of pleasure. Pleasure can mean different things at different times. Perhaps you're going to have a different kind of orgasm or you're going to try something new. When engaging in partner play, always remember:

- Your body merits respect and value.

- Your sexual interests deserve exploration.

- Your erotic actions are never to be shamed.

- Your boundaries are there to be honored.

- And your pleasure is worth everything.

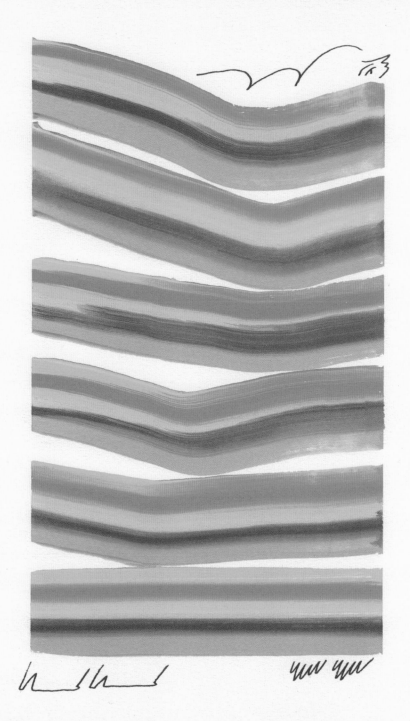

6

Final

Thoughts:

Be the

Person You

Need to See

When you feel good about your body, you feel good about your choices. And when you feel good about your choices, you can feel good about your pleasure.

My dearest reader,

When you first started this book, where were you in your pleasure-seeking life? Was it nonexistent? Did you have uninhibited sexy moments? Were you present in your pleasure? Go back to the beginning and check in on the note that you wrote.

Throughout this journey, I've asked you so many questions. I've challenged you to consider yourself before others. I've laid out rituals, practices, and various ways to connect to your pleasure. And now look where you are: You have come to a deeper understanding of how you operate in this world, in your body, in relationships, and in bed. You are the true master of your pleasure sphere. You've come a long way, reader. You should really be so proud of yourself.

Now that you're here, it's time for you to take what you've learned and apply it to your day-to-day life. Your pleasure is an integral part of your happiness. Not only will it reinforce the love you have for yourself, but it can also inspire others around you to begin their journey.

You are the true master of your pleasure sphere.

Of course, not every day can we take a step back and live life to its peak pleasure (your job, your responsibilities—those aren't going anywhere). Inevitably, there are going to be bad days, days when pleasure isn't your top priority. But instead of throwing your hands up and letting others dictate your circumstances, you now have the tools to guide your actions:

- Cry. Let it out.

- Breathe. Find that calm within your body.

- Be kind—to yourself and to others.

- Remember and act on your pleasures.

- Nourish your body with food you love.

- Do a little stretch.

- Find solace in your own masturbatorium.

- Write down what you're feeling.

- Go for a walk.

- Call a friend.

- Watch your favorite show.

- Take a few moments before acting on anything.

Today, however, is a good day because you've gotten here. And while this is the end of *My Pleasure*, it is just the beginning of your pleasure-filled life.

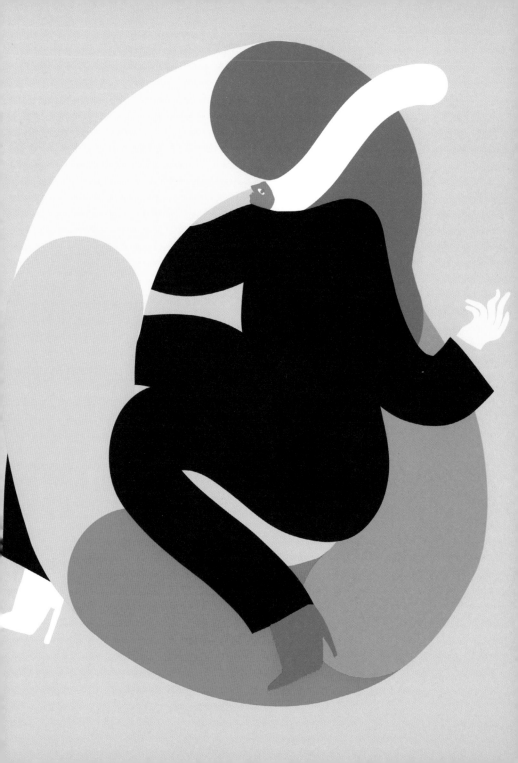

Sex, your body, your IRL, and every decision you make are so deeply connected. You are the 9 a.m. conference call and the 9 p.m. masturbation session. The way you see and treat yourself flows into everything you touch and then right back to you. Living a pleasurable life and giving yourself pleasure expands your self-love. Self-love means more empathy for yourself, more acknowledgment of your decisions, more confidence—plus really, really, really hot sex with yourself and with the lucky people you allow to touch your delicious body.

Love your body. Love yourself. Embrace your pleasure.

Thank you for going on this journey with me.

Remember: Above all else, you deserve pleasure and a pleasurable life.

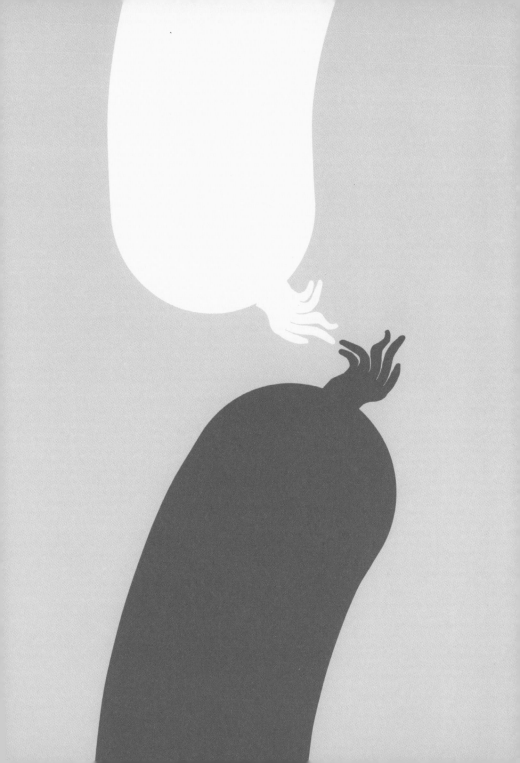

Glossary

ABSTINENCE: The choice to not engage in sexual interactions, and an absolutely fine choice to make over your own body.

ADVOCATE: A person who calls attention to a social problem and actively works toward positive change to address the problem. This can also mean being an advocate for yourself.

AFTERCARE: The emotional, physical, and spiritual care that one partner provides another partner after a sexual or intimate encounter.

AGE PLAY: A form of role-playing in which one person consensually acts or treats another as if they were a different age, whether in a sexual or nonsexual context.

ANAL: The stimulation of the anus through touch, rubbing, licking (a.k.a. analingus), penetrating, or plugging. It can be done by anyone for anyone of any sexual orientation or gender.

ANALINGUS: The sexual stimulation involving oral contact with the anus.

BALLS: Also known as testicles or testes, the balls are two organs that hang from a pouch of skin called the scrotum, which attaches to the shaft of the penis. The balls are incredibly sensitive and respond to light touch and licking with consent.

BDSM: An acronym used to describe sexual, sensual, intimate, and power relationships that derive from the following categories: bondage and discipline, domination and submission, sadism and masochism.

BLOW JOB: This is a slang term for oral sex on a person with a penis.

BODY IMAGE: The internal image a person has about their own body. It's influenced by the person's self-esteem.

BODY NEUTRALITY: The idea that a person should focus on what their body can do rather than what it looks like.

BODY POSITIVITY: A movement dedicated to empowering plus-size people and amplifying their experiences in a fatphobic society.

BONDAGE: The consensual practice of tying, binding, or restraining a partner for erotic, aesthetic, or somatosensory stimulation. This is also the *B* in *BDSM*.

BOOBS: A slang term for breasts. These can be rubbed, touched, grabbed, or massaged with consent.

BOTTOM: The receiving partner during sexual activity.

CAPACITY TO CONSENT: Refers to a person's ability to understand and make decisions; often connected to medical services or sexual encounters.

CASUAL SEX: Often described as having sex without emotional attachment, but there is emotion in being respectful; a sexual or intimate interaction with someone that a person emotionally respects outside of the bounds of a committed relationship.

COMMUNICATION: Sending or receiving information or conveying meanings from one entity or group to another.

CONSENSUAL NONCONSENT: This type of BDSM play is when everyone involved agrees to behave in a manner that mimics nonconsent and can involve impact play, psychological play, or pain and pleasure play. It requires a great deal of trust. Safe words, communication, and a deep level of understanding are all required in order to play at this level.

CONSENT: Agreeing to an action or a behavior. Consent occurs when one person voluntarily agrees to the proposal or desires of another. Consent is deeply important and a must for all sexual and human interactions.

CUMMING: Also known as an orgasm, that is, climax of sexual excitement, characterized by feelings of pleasure centered in the genitalia but can also spread to other parts of the body.

CUNNILINGUS: The act of orally stimulating the vulva and/or vagina.

DESIRE: A strong feeling of wanting to have something or wishing for something to happen.

DISCIPLINE: The practice where the dominant sets rules in which the submissive is expected to obey. This is also the *D* in *BDSM*.

DOM/DOMINANT: The partner who is controlling.

DOMINATION: This refers to when one partner exercises physical and/or emotional control over the other in both a sexual and nonsexual context. Note: Everyone involved needs to consent to take on this action. This is also the *D* in *BDSM*.

EMOTIONAL MATURITY: Managing one's emotions and responses to a tough scenario.

EROGENOUS ZONE: Parts of the body that stir sexual feelings or excitement when touched.

EXHIBITIONISM: The act of exposing one's body in a public or semipublic context.

FACE-SITTING: A sexual act in which one partner sits on or over the other's face, typically to allow or consensually force oral pleasure of the genitalia. Also known as queening or kinging.

FANTASY: Acting out or imagining a sexual or erotic scenario.

FAT: A fuel source for the body, a storage form of energy in the body, or having fat on the body. It's not a feeling—that is, a person cannot feel fat.

FETISH: An attraction to an object, such as an item of clothing or a part of the body.

FISTING: A sexual act where a person inserts their entire hand or fist into the other partner's vagina or anus—with consent and tons of lube.

GENDER IDENTITY: One's internal sense of their actual gender. This may be different from the gender they are perceived as by society and may be incongruent with the expectations of gender based on biological sex or culture. There are many different gender identities and it is important for people to self-identify their own rather than to be categorized against their will.

GROUP SEX: When three or more people engage in sex together. This could entail multiple people in the same room having consensual sex with particular partners, or having sex with everyone. Note: This is a very normal and fun way to experience pleasure with others.

HARD NO: A firm boundary around a feeling or an action that will not be changed.

IMPACT PLAY: An act where one person is struck by another person for erotic, sexual, power, or emotional gratification.

INDULGENCE: Actions that are an escape from the world we're in that don't consider the long-term benefits of our physical and emotional well-being.

INNER SABOTEUR: The part of the psyche or voice in one's head that operates based on fear and can sabotage real-life actions, plans, and aspirations.

INTIMACY: Closeness of one or more people in a caring, loving, platonic, or sexual relationship.

KINGING: A sexual act in which one partner sits on or over the other's face, typically to allow or consensually force oral pleasure of the genitalia. Also known as face-sitting or queening.

KINK: Refers to consensual, nontraditional sexual, sensual, and intimate behaviors such as sadomasochism, domination and submission, erotic role-playing, fetishism, and erotic forms of discipline.

LOUD SEX: Being super loud or screaming while you're having sex. If you're into it, great. If not, don't feel the need to perform. And if you have roommates or thin walls, turn up that Spotify playlist and go forth, babes!

LOVER: A sexual or romantic partner who could be in a casual or committed relationship with its own template.

LUBRICATION: A body-safe lubricant minimizes friction and allows smooth movement in or around orifices.

MAKING SPACE: Being physically, mentally, and emotionally present for another person to support them as they feel their feelings. Also called holding space.

MASOCHISM/MASOCHIST: The sexual gratification when enduring physical pain or humiliation. Note: Everyone involved needs to consent to take on this action. This is also the *M* in *BDSM*.

MASTURBATION: Also known as solo play or solo sex. This is having sex with yourself, and it is deeply pleasurable.

NAME-CALLING: The act of using pet or derogatory names during play to stir up an emotion or arousal.

ORGASM: A climax of sexual excitement, characterized by feelings of pleasure centered in the genitalia but can also spread to other parts of the body.

ORGY: A group of people who engage in sex with multiple partners in a single sitting or scene.

PEGGING: A person with a penis being penetrated anally for sexual gratification. Often in reference to heterosexual couples.

PLAY: The activities that take place in a sexual encounter, an intimate moment, or a BDSM scene.

PLAY PARTY: A social event where attendees socialize and engage in BDSM and sexual activities together.

PLEASURE: A state of gratification, a sensual gratification, a frivolous amusement. Pleasure enhances the life we are building, not escaping from.

POWER DYNAMICS/POWER EXCHANGE: The exchange of power between groups or people, which can be a useful tool in consensual role-playing.

QUEENING: A sexual act in which one partner sits on or over the other's face, typically to allow or consensually force oral pleasure of the genitalia. Also known as face-sitting or kinging.

ROLE-PLAY: Acting out or performing the part of a person or character during an erotic or sexual experience. This is a great time to introduce power dynamics into the play.

ROUGH SEX: Very vigorous sex with elements of pain (spanking, slapping, etc.).

SADISM/SADIST: A person who receives sexual gratification from causing pain and degradation to another. Note: Everyone involved needs to consent to take on this action. This is also the *S* in *BDSM*.

SCENE: A preplanned setting and space where a BDSM activity will take place.

SELF-ACCEPTANCE: The awareness and acceptance of one's strengths and weaknesses.

SELF-AWARENESS: The conscious knowledge of one's own character, feelings, motives, and desires.

SELF-CARE: The action a person takes to be mindful of their own needs, such as getting enough rest, drinking water, minimizing stress, having a wellness regimen, and performing beauty rituals.

SELF-ESTEEM: The confidence in one's abilities and worth.

SEX: The sexual activity between one or multiple consenting partners using inter-, outer-, or any kind of course that works for the people involved.

SEX PLAYLIST: A series of music played to help you get in the mood.

SEX POSITIVITY: A stance toward human sexuality that regards all consensual sexual activities as healthy and pleasurable.

SEX TOYS: An object or a device used for sexual stimulation or to enhance sexual pleasure.

SLAPPING: The act of hitting or striking with the palm of the hand or a flat object. Note: Participants must ensure consent and that the impact occurs on a safe area of the body—noting there is always an inherent risk to impact play.

SLUT: A person who knows what they want sexually. Often used as a derogatory term for someone who likes to have sex or is outspoken about sex, but not at all a shameful moniker and should be ignored if used in a pejorative manner.

SPANKING: The act of striking another person on different body parts—most notably on the buttocks—for sexual arousal or gratification.

SQUIRTING: When a person with a vulva ejaculates during sexual stimulation.

STRAP-ON SEX: Sex that involves using a prosthetic phallus for oral, vaginal, or anal sex, dry humping, or masturbation. Strap-on sex can occur between those of any gender or sexual orientation but always with consenting adults.

SUB/SUBMISSIVE: The partner who is being controlled.

SUBMISSION: A set of sexual rituals and behaviors in which a person willingly yields control of their bodies to a dominating force or the will of another person when acting out a sexual fantasy or any erotic behavior, and requires consent. This is also the *S* in *BDSM*.

SWITCH: A person who is comfortable in either the submissive role or the dominant role.

TOP: The partner who performs the sexual or erotic action, or who gives or penetrates during sexual activity. (But this also brings up a larger question: Is the person performing a blow job the top or bottom?)

VANILLA SEX: Sex that lacks a kink element, but not at all boring, as it is often perceived to be.

VOYEURISM: The sexual pleasure from watching others when they are naked or during sexual activity.

WATER SPORTS: The act of urinating on another person or watching someone urinate for sexual arousal. Politicians deny doing it. People make jokes about it. Shame ensues for those interested in it. It can be tied into domination play.

YES/NO/MAYBE LIST: A list of sexual, sensual, and intimate actions that can be used as a tool to communicate with a sexual partner.

Resources

BOOKS

Allen, Samantha. *Real Queer America: LGBT Stories from Red States.* New York: Little, Brown and Company, 2019.

Chase, Ella. *Curvy Girl Sex: 101 Body-Positive Positions to Empower Your Sex Life.* Beverly, MA: Fair Winds Press, 2017.

Comella, Lynn. *Vibrator Nation: How Feminist Sex-Toy Stores Changed the Business of Pleasure.* Durham, NC: Duke University Press, 2017.

Davina, Lola. *Thriving in Sex Work: Heartfelt Advice for Staying Sane in the Sex Industry.* Oakland, CA: The Erotic as Power Press, 2017.

Dionne, Evette. *Fat Girls Deserve Fairy Tales Too: Living Hopefully on the Other Side of Skinny.* New York: Basic Books, 2020.

Gordon, Aubrey. *What We Don't Talk about When We Talk about Fat.* Boston: Beacon Press, 2020.

Holliday, Tess. *The Not So Subtle Art of Being a Fat Girl: Loving the Skin You're In.* Richmond, CA: Weldon Owen, 2017.

Horn, Tina. *SFSX (SAFE SEX).* Portland, Oregon: Image Comics, 2020.

Katz, Anne. *Sex When You're Sick: Reclaiming Sexual Health after Illness or Injury.* Westport, CT: Praeger, 2009.

Ligon, Zoë. *Carnal Knowledge: Sex Education You Didn't Get in School.* Munich: Prestel, 2020.

Naphtali, Kate, Edith MacHattie, and Stacy Elliott. *PleasureABLE: Sexual Device Manual for Persons with Disabilities.* Vancouver: Disabilities Health Research Network, 2009.

Newport, Jerry and Mary Newport. *Autism-Asperger's and Sexuality: Puberty and Beyond.* Arlington, TX: Future Horizons, 2002.

Patterson, Kevin A. *Love's Not Color Blind: Race and Representation in Polyamorous and Other Alternative Communities.* Portland, OR: Thorntree Press, 2018.

Rothman, Julia, and Shaina Feinberg. *Every Body: An Honest and Open Look at Sex from Every Angle.* New York: Voracious, 2021.

Strings, Sabrina. *Fearing the Black Body: The Racial Origins of Fat Phobia.* New York: New York University Press, 2019.

Taylor, Sonya Renee. *The Body Is Not an Apology: The Power of Radical Self-Love.* Oakland, CA: Berrett-Koehler Publishers, 2018.

Tobia, Jacob. *Sissy: A Coming-of-Gender Story.* New York: G. P. Putnam's, 2019.

Tovar, Virgie. *The Self-Love Revolution: Radical Body Positivity for Girls of Color.* Oakland, CA: Instant Help Books, 2020.

Tovar, Virgie. *You Have the Right to Remain Fat.* New York: Feminist Press, 2018.

Vernon, Leah. *Unashamed: Musings of a Fat, Black Muslim.* Boston: Beacon Press, 2019.

Yeboah, Stephanie. *Fattily Ever After: A Black Fat Girl's Guide to Living Life Unapologetically.* London: Hardie Grant, 2020.

PODCASTS

Find these wherever you get your podcasts:

Balanced Black Girl

Big Calf

Disarming Disability

Food 4 Thot

Future of Sex

Girls on Porn

Hear to Slay

Inner Hoe Uprising

Loving BDSM

Maintenance Phase

Sex with Emily

She's All Fat

Where Should We Begin?

Why Are People into That?!

Why Won't You Date Me?

NEWSLETTERS

The Audacity by Roxane Gay / audacity.substack.com

The Bottom's Line by Chingy Nea / thegaychingy.substack.com

Fran's Joy Digest by Fran Tirado / fransquishco.substack.com

In-Box by Bobby Box / bobbybox.substack.com

Salty / saltyworld.net

Pleasure Pie / Pleasurepie.org

ONLINE RESOURCES

Ask a Sub / An online resource for submissives askasub.com

Bex Talks Sex / Yes, No, Maybe List bextalkssex.com/yes-no-maybe/

Glamputee / Alex Locust's guides to disability justice and microaggressions. glamputee.com/resources

Hey Epiphora / Queer-inclusive sex toy reviews heyepiphora.com

Kinky: The Documentary / A funny, informational look at Black sexuality and the BDSM community. https://vimeo.com/414266410

Lesbian Herstory Archives / Records detailing Lesbian lives for future generations. Lesbianherstoryarchives.org

MakeLoveNotPorn / A social sex video sharing platform. Makelovenotporn.tv

Sugarbutch / Toy reviews, dirty stories, workshops sugarbutch.net

Thick Str1p Enterprises / Body Positive Strip Show instagram.com/thickstripent

SEX TOY COMPANIES AND ACCESSORIES MANUFACTURERS

Aneros / aneros.com

b-Vibe / bvibe.com

Babeland / babeland.com

Bellesa Boutique / bboutique.co

The Cowgirl / ridethecowgirl.com

Dame / dameproducts.com

enby / shopenby.com

Gnat / gnat.shop

Le Wand / lewandmassager.com

LeatherCoven / etsy.com/shop/leathercoven

New York Toy Collective / newyorktoycollective.com

njoy / njoytoys.com

Ohnut / ohnut.co

Please / pleasenyc.com

The Pleasure Chest / thepleasurechest.com

Plume / houseofplume.com

Sliquid / sliquid.com

SpareParts HardWear / myspare.com

Spectrum Boutique / spectrumboutique.com

Tantus / tantusinc.com

Tenga / tenga.co

Unbound / unboundbabes.com

Vixen Creations / vixen-creations.myshopify.com

We-Vibe / we-vibe.com

PORN AND EROTICA

Aurore / readaurore.com

Best Women's Erotica of the Year / bweoftheyear.com

Crashpad / crashpadseries.com

Dipsea / dipseastories.com

Eros / eros.110west40th.com

Math Magazine / mathmagazine.com

Peach Fuzz / peachfuzzmag.com

BODY, GENDER, AND SEX POSITIVE ORGANIZATIONS

BIPOC Adult Industry Collective / bipoc-collective.org

Fat Girls Travel Too / fatgirlstraveltoo.com

The Gender Unicorn / transstudent.org/gender

Kink and Poly Aware Professionals Directory (KAP) / kapprofessionals.org

National Center for Transgender Equality / transequality.org

Sex Down South Conference / sexdownsouth.com

Trans Women of Color Collective / twocc.us

THERAPY PROFESSIONALS AND ORGANIZATIONS

American Association of Sexuality Educators, Counselors and Therapists / aasect.org

Ashlee Bennet / bodyimage-therapist.com

Cameron Glover / info.cameronglover.com

Casey W. Tanner / queer-therapy.com

Donna Oriowo / annodright.com/drdonnaoriowo

Heather Irobunda /irobundamd.com

Joy Cox / drjoycox.com

Julia Greco / juliagreco.com

Kimbritive / kimbritive.com

Nedra Glover Tawwab / nedratawwab.com

Radical Therapy Center / radicaltherapycenter.com

Raquel Savage / raquelsavage.com

Rosa Sierra / msha.ke/sexandempathy

Shadeen Francis / shadeenfrancis.com

Sonalee Rashatwar, The Fat Sex Therapist / sonaleer.com

Tasha Bailey / realtalktherapist.co.uk

Acknowledgments

Thank you to the babes with the best hearts who made space for me to try, fail, succeed, fail some more, and start all over again in order to find my path: Grandma, Aunt Roe, Dana, Gina, Antoinette, Hannah, Amber. Kelly, Jill and Blanche, Heather, Sophia: I'll never be able to thank you enough.

Thank you to the Chronicle team for the love and care it took to bring this book together: Claire, Sydney, Rachel, Magnolia, Maddie, and Cynthia.

Erika, your undying support has made this all possible.

Isabelita, you're my North Star no matter where we are.

To anyone who has ever felt like they didn't deserve more, this is for you.

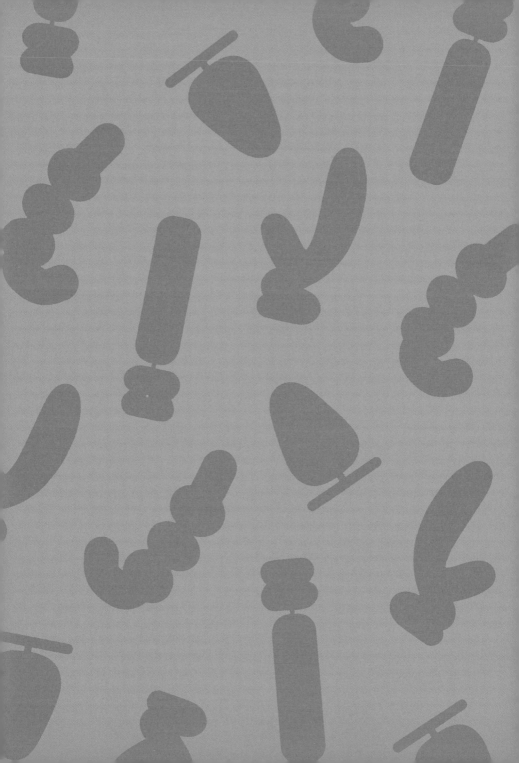